W9-BLP-420

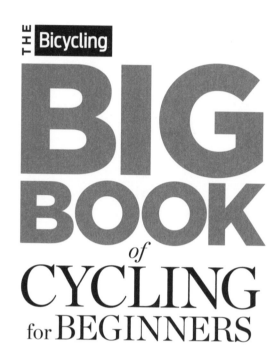

THE Bicycling
BIG BOOK
BOOK
of
CYCLING
for BEGINNERS

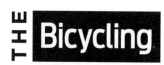

BIG BOOK

of

CYCLING

for BEGINNERS

**Everything a New Cyclist Needs to Know
to Gear Up and Start Riding**

TORI BORTMAN

Notice: The information in this book is meant to supplement, not replace, proper exercise training. All forms of exercise pose some inherent risks. The editors and publisher advise readers to take full responsibility for their safety and know their limits. Before practicing the exercises in this book, be sure that your equipment is well-maintained, and do not take risks beyond your level of experience, aptitude, training, and fitness. The exercise and dietary programs in this book are not intended as a substitute for any exercise routine or dietary regimen that may have been prescribed by your doctor. As with all exercise and dietary programs, you should get your doctor's approval before beginning.

Mention of specific companies, organizations, or authorities in this book does not imply endorsement by the author or publisher, nor does mention of specific companies, organizations, or authorities imply that they endorse this book, its author, or the publisher.

Internet addresses and telephone numbers given in this book were accurate at the time it went to press.

© 2014 by Rodale Inc.

Photographs © 2014 by Rodale, except: 19, 33, 53, 86, 91, 97, 115, 117, 119, 151, 205, 228, 229, 233, 234, 236, 240, 241 ©Daniel Sharp; 7a ©Tom Bol; 7b ©Jordan Siemans; 7c ©Paul Elledge; 9 ©Charles Gullung; 13 ©Getty Images; 56 ©Braxton Bruce; 82 ©Michael Robertson; 93 ©Adam Hester; 109 ©Embry Rucker; 110 ©Douglas Benedict; 111 ©Francois Portman; 114 ©Michael Robertson; 128 ©Technotr/Getty Images; 131 ©Bryce Boyer; 158 ©Angie Smith; 213 ©Getty Images; 188b ©Brand X Pictures

Photography on 29, 73, 226, 227 by Mitch Mandel; 35, 66, 83, 188a, 188c by Thomas MacDonald.

Illustrations © 2014 by Adam Wallenta

All rights reserved. No part of this publication may be reproduced or transmitted in any form or by any means, electronic or mechanical, including photocopying, recording, or any other information storage and retrieval system, without the written permission of the publisher.

Rodale books may be purchased for business or promotional use or for special sales. For information, please write to: Special Markets Department, Rodale, Inc., 733 Third Avenue, New York, NY 10017

Bicycling is a registered trademark of Rodale Inc.

Printed in the United States of America

Rodale Inc. makes every effort to use acid-free ∞, recycled paper ♻.

Book design by Joanna Williams

Library of Congress Cataloging-in-Publication Data
is on file with the publisher.

978-1-62336-164-8

Distributed to the trade by Macmillan

2 4 6 8 10 9 7 5 3 1   paperback

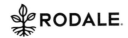

We inspire and enable people to improve their lives and the world around them.
rodalebooks.com

For my students, who remind me to live with the wonder,
curiosity, and openness of a beginner's mind and
that true courage comes not from strength or knowledge,
but from vulnerability and leaps of faith.

Contents

Introduction

THERE ARE MANY, MANY REASONS TO START ROAD CYCLING, but usually it comes down to something that's drawing you to it. It could be that you'd like to regain some of the wonder of childhood in a more grown-up way. Maybe you get a jealous twinge hearing about your brother-in-law's epic weekend rides. Sometimes it's the sit-down, dead-serious talk your doctor gives you about your health that's making you see the potential of pavement for the first time.

In reality, it doesn't matter what called you here, only that you've decided to heed it. Welcome. You're in for a fun ride.

Simplicity in Action

Bikes haven't really changed much since their inception. They are essentially still just two wheels, a chain, and our momentum keeping us in balance. Most of the big gains in cycling technology have come by way of making the bike more comfortable so we can spend more time in the saddle. Otherwise, it's pretty much the same machine we learned on as kids, but easier and more comfortable to ride.

The beauty of the road bike is that it doesn't ask for much. It doesn't tell you why or when to ride. It's there waiting patiently if you decide to hop in the saddle and is not hurt when you walk by and hop in your car to head for work. It doesn't say "you're not fast enough" or give you guff for not being first to the top of the hill. It can be the perfect companion.

The simple motion of cycling has a funny way of making things clearer, less cluttered, a little slower, and a bit more real. Whether you're speeding toward a finish line or cruising on a weeklong bike tour, it connects you to the present moment—the here and now—in a way that most things in our fast-paced, high-tech world can't. It helps bring awareness to the small things—the temperature of the air, the subtle changes in terrain—making real connections to the world around you.

Freedom

For most of us, riding our first bike was a rite of passage: the electric rush of happiness when we rode on our own and really spread our wings for the first time. Bikes gave us the independence and courage to go around the block, to the store, and farther and farther away into our own adventures.

Now in our adulthood, we're often just not convinced we can ever get that feeling back. The secret is, being on the road on your bike, listening to your breath, and pushing the pedals is pretty much the same as it was back then. It's a very low-tech getaway car.

Most road cyclists will describe "sneaking away for a ride" or "letting it go on the pavement." Being on the bike is just you, the

pavement, and ribbons of white and yellow lines. For the first time you can shake the day off and look up—really look up—and see the beauty of the world around you.

Road cycling is a means to an end. It's one way we can ride away from the phone, the house, the bills, the TV, what's going on at work, how the kids are driving you bonkers. Getting on the bike is the antidote. It's a mini-vacation for your soul. It's a time to revamp and breathe—even if it's just for an hour at a time.

Sneaking Up on Your Confidence

Although getting on the bike is simple, we're unlikely to have the grace or strength of a professional racer. There's a lot to learn, and this book will help guide you.

The cool thing is that with every new skill—from becoming a graceful descender to being able to easily grab your water bottle without bobbling—your confidence on the bike will grow. Confidence is a funny thing. Almost like a virus, it can affect your whole life, your well-being, and even those around you. Right now you may see yourself as someone who just wants to get into better shape. It's likely you'll get there before you know it, and when you see how easy it is to reach one goal, it will be easier to set and accomplish another—one that may not even be on the bike.

It starts with the hill you never thought you'd

The Myth of the Elite

ROAD CYCLING HAS A LONG AND CHERISHED history of being the sport of godlike men who gutted themselves climbing frozen mountain passes and endured the heat of a thousand deserts to come to be the first to cross a finish line. There is a tiny speck of truth to the myth. No doubt, these riders are impressive and have accomplished great feats.

This notion, which is intended to motivate, sometimes alienates new riders. Road cycling has typically been viewed as a "get epic or get out" show of suffering and ego. If we aren't the kind of men or women who want to go after every goal as if it's a matter of life and death, then it's easy to get the impression that road cycling isn't for us mere "mortals." Races like the Tour de France can be a source of inspiration and a testament to the strength of the human spirit, but they can often leave the rest of us feeling left out of the cycling "club"—as if we will never have cool-enough clothes or state-of-the-art bicycles, and as if we will never be fast enough to really fit in.

Luckily the cycling world has mostly outgrown the idea that you can't get on a road bike unless you have something to prove, the fastest bike, and the trimmest physique. The thin threads holding together the "elite club" fabrication have worn out, and one and all are now welcome to experience the joy of the open road.

As a sport, cycling started as a new way for every man—and in groundbreaking ways, every woman—to get around quickly and be liberated on the road. It became a great equalizer, and, lucky for us, road cycling is now enjoying a renaissance as it is reclaimed by everyday people. There is no horde of spandex-clad riders waiting to make fun of you for not being fast or cool or strong enough. You can ride confidently no matter what your skill level is or what you're wearing or how long it's been since you were last on a bike. Everyone is now welcome, no experience or particular grit required.

Just bring a curiosity of what the road ahead holds and the desire to have a memorable time getting there, and let the good times roll.

be able to climb, which eventually becomes the hill you never thought you'd be able to climb without stopping, which then finally becomes the hill that you conquer with ease. That kind of progression in the saddle can also help you wrap your mind around asking for that long overdue raise or realize that dream of starting your own business. You'll learn what it's like to try, fall short of your goals, and keep trying

again knowing you'll eventually get where you want to go.

Health

Health benefits seem like a no-brainer. You're going to get fit, right? Maybe lose a few pounds while you're at it? Cycling is a good way to control your weight, but whether you shed pounds or not, you'll still be getting big payouts. The cardiovascular workout that cycling provides can not only help control diabetes, prevent heart disease, lower your blood pressure, and put you at a lower risk for cancer, but it can also increase your overall muscle strength and endurance so you can do more of the other things you already love, and they'll likely get easier.

With this comes a lot of other great benefits—including boosting your brainpower and your sex drive while lowering your stress levels. If that's not enough, it can boost your immunity as well. So when your friends start asking what's gotten you into this new cycling habit, you can smile and honestly say, "I just feel so much better."

Calories in = Pedaling out

Road cycling will likely help you drop some weight, especially if you're coming to it from a not very active lifestyle. Because a lot of people get hooked on riding, they find themselves in the saddle more and more. Of course, you'll also be eating on the bike, which will even things out a bit. But oftentimes cycling changes your relationship to food for the better.

Whereas before you ate because it was time to eat, now you might find yourself eating to fuel your rides. As you slim down, your speed and your self-esteem will go up. Of course for most cyclists, we also use cycling as a great excuse to eat our favorite treats. Whether it's beer or chocolate chip cookies, you can reward yourself for a job well done.

Boosting Your Brain

When you start pedaling your bike there are a lot of physical reactions going on. You heart beats faster, your lungs take in fuller breaths, your muscles contract, and your digestive system kicks in. The cool part is, all those physical reactions have a mental counterpart as well.

As you increase fitness, the part of your brain that controls long-term and spatial memory consequently grows as well. In older adults, exercise can stave off Alzheimer's. Because cycling requires balance, instantaneous decision-making skills, and quick reaction time, you'll be better at solving puzzles (including those stubborn life problems that always seem to be creeping up).

Some studies have shown that vigorous exercise can help alleviate depression, anxiety, and even attention deficit disorder—and sometimes prevent them from happening in the first place.

Sexual Healing

There is an unfortunate urban myth going around that cycling can decrease your pleasure or performance in the bedroom. Luckily, nothing can be further from the truth. That sweet aerobic workout on your road bike has a direct correlation to increased stamina in other arenas—including in bed.

First off, regular exercise increases our testosterone production. It's important to note that this little hormone makes you want to pursue, initiate, and have sex. Who couldn't use a little more of that? Not to mention getting fit and active has been shown to increase the frequency of arousal, function, satisfaction, and—by up to a 30 percent increase—sexual activity.

In one study of female cyclists at the University of Texas at Austin, cycling was found to help increase arousal in women right after a ride—both emotionally and physically (with more bloodflow to their lady parts).

In 2003 research by the Harvard School of Public Health found that men over 50 who were physically active were not only less likely to suffer from erectile dysfunction, but some had the performance of men up to 5 years younger. Those are the kind of results that make it worth getting in the saddle.

Bicycling

BIG
BOOK
of
CYCLING
for BEGINNERS

PART I

FINDING THE RIGHT RIDE FOR YOU

You want to ride a bike on the road, plain and simple, right? But knowing where you're going is the first step to getting there. In this often overwhelming, have-it-your-way culture, there are a lot of choices in road bikes, so it's helpful to narrow things down by examining your aspirations before you get started. The kind of riding you want to do will have a huge influence on what kind of bike you should buy. We'll help you get a better idea of the types of rides the road offers and which ones interest you the most. Maybe we'll even inspire you to dream up new adventures that hadn't been on your radar. There's a lot of road to explore out there, and a lot of ways to experience it!

WHATCHA GONNA DO?

You may not think you have big dreams when it comes to getting on the road. How about some simple expectations of how you'll perform, where you'll go, or how fast you'll get there? When you articulate what you want (and, just as importantly, what you don't), your time on the road can be thrilling and gratifying rather than frustrating or disappointing. In other words, you won't be kicking yourself for using the broad stroke of "road riding" to invest in a race bike when all you really want is to comfortably ride with a few friends—and maybe occasional sprints to the sign for the county line.

The types of cyclists putting rubber to pavement and their riding styles are wildly varied, from Lycra-clad racers to wool-bedecked club riders. In fact, once you start riding, you may find you want to overlap into one or more of these categories. As you read this section, prioritize how much time or how often you'll be riding, as well as what type of riding you might want to do. This is also a helpful primer on the different types of cycling groups you may encounter on the road that will give you a little perspective on how the other side pedals and perhaps open your mind to new possibilities of where the pavement can lead you.

CHAPTER 1

Just Rolling Along: The Recreational Rider

YOU DON'T WANT TO COMPETE, AND LOSING A FEW POUNDS might be a bonus, but you're attracted to bicycling as an experience. Maybe you'd like to explore the world around you a little more closely, or find a way to spend time with friends (or make new ones) on two wheels. You foresee days when you may want to get there fast, but most days you're just happy to be on the bike making the wheels spin and taking the world in stride. If these characteristics sum up your cycling attitude, then recreational riding is a great fit for you.

Why Recreational Riding Might Be Calling You

Although all types of road riding are enjoyable, recreational riding is defined as riding "just for the joy of it." This is how a lot of people get hooked on road riding, a gateway drug of sorts. For some it's a gentle entry into the sport end of cycling. That's not to say everyone upgrades to racing from here. If you blanch at the word "training," this type of riding is probably where you want to start exploring the road—you'll usually be pedaling at your pace, and your ability to meander will be limited only by your imagination.

Recreational riding is the one type of road riding that also tends to encourage indulgence. These rides often start and end at cafés, sometimes with an unhurried lunch stop in the middle. Got a late start? When riding for pleasure, it's okay to roll out whenever you please. The pushing of pedals in this case is to savor the sights and sounds around you, find the less-traveled path, and make new connections to the land and the people in it.

Recreational riding experience is often—but not always—a social one. Not that you won't make friends when fitness riding or racing, but in those cases you're often breathing too hard to chat or timing and routing get in the way. Recreational riding lends itself to the companionship and camaraderie that come with the pursuit of leisure. When done in groups, these are "no drop" rides where riders stick together because that's exactly the point: to have a good time, together.

All that being said, this type of riding doesn't have to be done in groups at all. It can be a day on the bike with no destination, or a day when the goal is a far-flung quirky landmark. It can mean solo touring—adventuring off into the wild to explore new territory. Even if you're commuting or cycle touring on your own, you're bound to meet and connect with more people along the way than you would during other types of cycling.

What Recreational Riding Looks Like

Whether solo or in a group, this riding is all about the experience, recapturing the joys of childhood, and taking stock of the world rolling by. Recreational riding is recess on a road bike—and there's no end to the games you can play.

Many riders of all stripes start by *riding solo*. Like a young fawn taking its first steps, sometimes the joy of getting there is enough. These riders find that they prefer to pedal along on their own, keeping their personal pace and timeline and enjoying the quiet time.

Riding with friends is the most common way to head out for a gratifying spin. These can be short rides on paved, off-road bike paths or endless meandering on back roads to the next town over—where you might even find yourself catching the bus back depending on how you're feeling. Imagine an impromptu pub crawl but instead of drinking beer at every pub, you nosh on doughnuts, tacos, or coffee at each stop. You can ride with friends for fitness or racing, but in both those cases, pedaling and how much your body gets out of it are the focus, rather than the company you keep or the destination.

Some riders prefer to ride as an organized group. One way to do this is to join a local *club ride*. Often volunteer-run bike clubs are free resources for riders to find rides and routes, with descriptions, events, support, clinics, and more. Most put on regularly scheduled weekly or monthly rides, some with predetermined routes. Cycling clubs and their ride schedules can be found either online or through your local bicycle shop.

Club rides are usually advertised at a designated speed and distance so you have an idea of how fast and far the ride will be, or they will split into "A" and "B" groups so riders can participate at a pace that feels best for them. To keep your ride fun, don't get in over your head with long distances from the jump. Most club rides have a "no drop" policy, meaning that no rider will be left behind. However, every cyclist is responsible for his or her own support— meaning you carry your own food and water, repair your own mechanical problems, and find a way back if the problem is too big to fix on the side of the road. Be aware that some clubs offer "race pace" or "training" rides, which won't be as social as the slower, recreational rides.

If you have questions about the rides, there is usually a contact person who is the main organizer and can offer details. Don't be too intimidated to ask questions. These clubs exist to foster and create new riders and cycling opportunities, so they want to help you. All club rides are usually open to the general public (meaning you don't have to become a member or pay dues to ride), and they are a great way to meet fellow riders and find new routes in your region.

Through clubs or on your own, you might find *event rides*. These are group rides on a much larger (anywhere from 200 to 2,000 participants) scale that take place over a few hours, or up to a week or more. The routes are often very beautiful or historically interesting, with locales that your regional bike club might not offer. These rides provide rest stops every 10 to 15 miles along the route with food and water, mechanical support, sag vehicles to pick up riders who for one reason or another don't make it along the way, and sometimes pre- and postride meals. The ride organizers might also throw in a T-shirt or pint glass as memorabilia of your experience. All event rides have an entrance fee that covers all that pampering, and some are fundraisers for a particular cause.

The longer *event rides* can last up to a week, include everything listed above, and also supply all meals, accommodations, transport of your luggage, and sometimes even a rental bike. In the United States, many states offer some type of weeklong ride like this. If you're looking for something a little more far flung, there are rides like this around the world that can give you a great taste of the local topography, culture, and, of course, cuisine. Some are even centered specifically on the cooking or wine of a specific region. What better way to connect to cyclists than through their stomachs?

Last but not least, *bicycle touring* is one of the most revered types of recreational riding by all types of riders. Road touring involves picking a point-to-point destination or a loop of roads, which you'll cover over a series of days. The big difference between this and any event ride is that you'll be carrying all your gear: food, clothes, water, repair kits, possibly a tent and sleeping bag—everything. This may seem overwhelming for some beginners, but for others it's an open invitation to newfound adventures.

It's good to start with a 2- to 3-day tour to get your legs under you and give you a sense of how far and fast you like to travel in a day. You can build up to traveling weeks or months at a time, exploring faraway countries or just getting to know your own on a whole new, more intimate level. Luckily, there are many resources out there for inspiration, routes, and travel advice for those wanting to explore on two wheels.

There are a few variations on this type of riding. You can go a little lighter weight with what you haul but heavier on expenses—the "credit card" tour—meaning you don't tote along your food or shelter and instead eat meals at restaurants and sleep at hotels or hostels. Another more adventurous and self-sustaining option is to carry all your supplies and camp along the way, and then stop at grocery stores as needed to re-up on supplies. This second choice frees up many more miles of pavement for the rider because he or she can journey outside of highly populated (and therefore possibly heavily trafficked) areas.

Another choice to consider is with whom, if anyone, you'd like to tour. The trick to finding good touring pals is knowing that you ride at approximately similar speeds and have decided roughly how often and how long you want to stop. This can go awry quickly if you have a stronger rider who prefers to plow through miles and a slower rider who prefers to stop often. Most touring guides suggest that the best way to tour is to focus on the recreational aspect, stop often to eat, and explore the land you're journeying through. If you can't (or don't want to) find someone to ride with, touring solo is both safe and a good time to get away from the hustle and bustle of the modern, plugged-in life.

Commuting (riding to work) and *everyday riding* (riding around town to run errands) are the last kinds of recreational riding.

You might question how commuting could be considered a "recreation." If you have the ability to cycle to work—meaning the stars align so that you live close enough to ride to work (20 miles or less) and you either have a job you can wear commuter gear to or your place of work offers facilities for you to clean up and change—it's one of the best ways to beat stress, get active, strengthen your immune system, get your brain revved up in the morning, and wind down on the way home. Much like touring, you'll need to carry a bit of gear, such as clothes to change into, maybe a laptop, and your lunch. Other than that, many riders come to find that getting to work by bicycle actually saves time

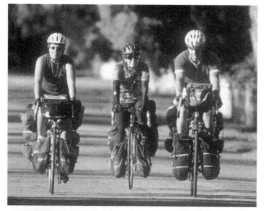

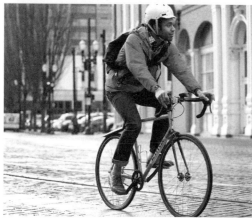

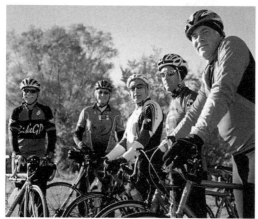

These three very different riders can all be considered "recreational" cyclists. Whether touring, commuting, or club riding, all are welcome.

off their commute, negates their gym membership, and leaves them happier and more productive on the job.

Commuting will likely put you on the roads with the heaviest motor vehicle traffic because of the times of day that you'll be traveling. If you're someone who feels nervous around cars and trucks, you have a few options. Most commuters avoid the routes that most cars would take and instead choose low-traffic side streets or bike paths and find other options that make the ride both safer and more enjoyable. Often this means discovering new parts of your neighborhood that you otherwise would have never ventured into. It's sometimes helpful to find a riding buddy from work who can help you find the easiest, fastest, and safest routes.

Everyday riding is similar to commuting but a good choice for individuals who don't have riding to work as an option. It's defined by accomplishing daily tasks, entertainment, and errands on two wheels. Your road bike can be a wonderful way to get to the library, grocery store, coffee shop, happy hour, or movie theater. You can even buy a trailer to cart your kids to school or to the park. Today the road bike can easily double as a utility bike, perfect for saving money on gas and enjoying some quality time on two wheels.

The same routing ideas apply to everyday riding as for commuting. Quiet side streets off the beaten path make for great cycling, and you'll need a good idea of how to navigate urban traffic. Otherwise, the sky is the limit on how far you can go or what you can carry. There have been entire households moved by bike using trailers, saddle bags, and backpacks to transport everything from the sofa and king-size bed to silverware, TVs, and coffee tables, so dream big!

What a Recreational Rider Looks Like

These are the hardest cyclists to pick out of a crowd because anyone—yes, anyone—can be a recreational road rider. It doesn't take a particular body type, fitness level, gender, or age. There are as many young riders using the bike as their way to get around as there are seniors adventuring around the globe. Depending on your comfort level (and how far you're going), you can do a lot of this pedaling in regular street clothes—no spandex required.

This is the cyclist that even friends or family may never know about—except for one detail: They are usually having such a great time on their bikes that they can't help but crow about it. Their secret is that there are no barriers to the escapades to be had or adventures imagined. Once you pursue the liberty a road bike can afford you, there really is no looking back.

The Recreation Bicycle(s)

Out of all the styles of road cycling, this bicycle gives you the most flexibility in budget and materials. That being said, there are a few things that most recreational bikes have in

Top Signs You Might Be a Recreational Rider

> ➤ The journey is more important than the destination.
> ➤ You never want to ride at a pace where you can't hold a conversation about the best coffee/bar/restaurant/bike shop in town.
> ➤ You like to go at your own pace.
> ➤ Your destinations are wild, curious, or sometimes completely arbitrary.
> ➤ Enjoying the scenery is a priority.
> ➤ If you had to get a ride home, you wouldn't feel a lick of shame.
> ➤ Training? What's training?
> ➤ You see road cycling as a great venue for socializing.
> ➤ You like other people to plan your rides and take care of all the details, like good food and stunning routes.
> ➤ You want to try camping by bike—maybe even totally self-sufficiently or solo.
> ➤ Sitting down and eating at a restaurant before, after, and/or during a ride sounds good to you.
> ➤ You want to see how much you can conceivably carry on a road bike.

common. Most recreational riders—but especially beginners—want a more upright position on the bike. This means that although you're still sitting in the traditional road position, less pressure will be on your hands and you'll have a better range of movement in your upper body to look around—for traffic or at the sights.

When day riding (which could be solo, with friends, a club ride, or an organized event), you can use the lightest, most high-tech machine or an ages-old ten-speed and still have a fantastic time. Truly, this type of riding encourages participation over products and gadgets. Other than always wearing your helmet, there's no

special gear required. On shorter rides and especially when commuting, you can ride in your jeans and a T-shirt with no worries about keeping up. As you progress to longer mileage, you'll find that you may want to invest in a few pieces of clothing that will make your ride a bit more comfortable, but when starting, you can really just jump right in.

The exception to this is self-supported cycle touring. Because you will need to haul at least a little gear, it's easiest with a bike that is built to accommodate a rack that you can hang bags from or strap gear onto. Of course, you can always opt to use the bike you have and haul a trailer, but if you're looking to buy your first

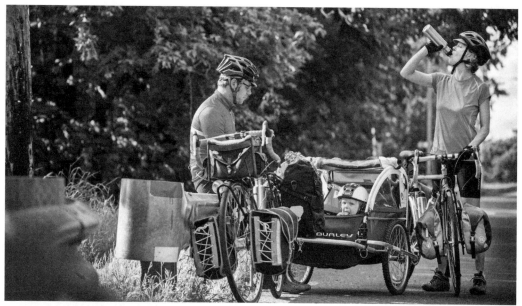

You can carry more than you'd imagine on a multiday tour.

bike, a touring bike is the chameleon of cycles. It can race, tour, commute, and is built extra tough so you can haul all the things you need. The bonus is that it's also extra durable—but with the downside of being the heaviest of all road bikes.

Recreational riders have one other option as well. There is a style of racing called "cyclo-cross," where the racers use a dropped-bar road bike that has wide, knobby tires and better clearance for mud. Commuter and cycle tourists also sometimes favor this type of bike because it offers good clearance for fenders and the ability to install racks. However, it has a smaller range of gearing choices, which some cycle tourists find limiting.

CHAPTER 2

Riding for a Healthier Life: The Fitness Cyclist

YOU LOOK AT A BIKE AND YOU SEE A WAY TO TEST YOUR BODY, get your heart pumping, and maybe lose a pound or two. You're not looking to race anybody . . . well, at least not right now, or maybe just your buddy up the next hill. You mostly want to spend time in the saddle getting fit and healthy, setting up personal goals and knocking them down.

Why Fitness Riding Might Be Calling You

Many people find themselves at a crossroads these days. On the one hand, it seems like so much work to get in shape—especially if you've never experienced any sort of athleticism. There are a lot of people who have never played sports, so they feel like cycling for exercise is a good, private place to start since you can do it alone and have your space—potentially not encountering anyone you know. Working out in a gym can seem both claustrophobic (being inside with loads of other sweaty people) and exhibitionist (rubbing sweaty elbows with the same folks 3 days a week)—not to mention it's hard to resist comparing yourself in that gym mirror, which can be an exercise in self-loathing.

Many people come to cycling as a way to make themselves healthier without the embarrassment or competition of other sports. You can head out on the road solo, or with a few supportive buddies. It's a common occurrence in bike shops that someone who has never been "fit," "athletic," or a participant in any sports outside of high school physical education walks in and buys a road bike. Since most of us—big or tall, hefty or thin, sporty or nerdy—have ridden a bike, it's an accessible and fun option for making ourselves healthier.

Some bike buyers find themselves heeding a doctor's warning that without some better choices, they're heading toward a lifetime of medication. For these individuals, fitness riding can be a solution and a savior.

Others have come from the doctor after their current activity has either caused or is causing too much damage to their bodies. Lifelong runners often find themselves hitting middle age with bad knees. Weekly "friendly" basketball games can wreak havoc on joints when middle age hits.

Or, it may not quite be time to give up your favorite activity yet, but you're looking for an opportunity to cross-train in another discipline.

One famed world-class motorcycle racer came to bicycling to build his cardio and mental endurance to condition him for moto race-day speeds of over 120 miles per hour. Finally, you might be inspired by the pro riders, with their machine-like endurance for altitude and pain. Every spring the men and women of the pro peloton bring themselves to the furthest reaches of their own capabilities. The alps they slay on the screen might be calling you to come test them yourself, but you have to start somewhere a little closer to home.

What a Fitness Ride Looks Like

As with any riding, this will vary from rider to rider. While cycling, the heart rate will be at a perceived exertion of somewhat hard to hard—an effort that feels hard but that you can maintain. If you've already got a solid athletic base, your first ride will be longer than if you're starting out fresh. Fitness riding is defined by the amount of time spent on the bike combined with the effort at which you're riding. Usually this type of rider will spend a minimum of an hour riding, working up to an average of an hour-and-a-half to more than 3 hours per ride, between 2 and 5 days a week.

This can be quite a time commitment, but it's also a great excuse to get away from the hurly-burly of our chaotic, plugged-in lives. This will also likely help you explore the place you live. You'll be branching out to the undiscovered, quiet, low-traffic roads surrounding you. There will be new places you've never seen and places you've seen that you'll observe in an entirely different light.

These rides usually take you outside of the city or on designated bike paths. If you're lucky enough to live in a more rural area, you can roll out from your door and spend less time stopping and starting at the stoplights that get you out of town.

Actual mileage will depend a lot on how fit you are, and even then how fast you are. Women often ride 2 to 3 miles per hour slower than men, even on their best days. So a 2-hour ride might take her 30 miles, while a man might be able to go closer to 40 miles. It all depends on the rider. Terrain and weather conditions will make a difference, too. A flat route might seem easier than a hilly one, but flat routes are also typically windier and not necessarily faster. In any case, most cyclists like to mix up their terrain.

What a Fitness Cyclist Looks Like

Funny thing about fitness riding—really any type of cycling—is that it's extremely forgiving. It's perhaps one of the most lenient sports you could choose to participate in—the opposite of

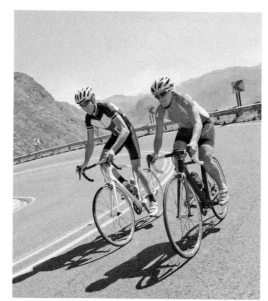

All body types are welcome, since fitness riding is what you make it.

a snobby clique. Bicycling will take anyone, of any age or body type. No tryouts, prerequisites, or age requirements.

The truth is, it *is* easier to climb hills the smaller you are. This is because of a better strength-to-weight ratio (medium + strong = fast, small + strong = faster). But larger riders descend faster and build more momentum to get up the next hill—and equally strong larger and smaller riders go nearly the same speed on flat ground.

As you begin your journey, play to your strengths. If your body helps you descend, then focus first on descending skills to give yourself a sense of accomplishment. After that, work on

Top Signs You Might Be a Fitness Rider

➤ You think Lycra looks silly, but if you were assured it made riding easier and more comfy, you'd buy some.

➤ In another land, far, far away, you used to be a runner/soccer player/swimmer/football player, but your shoulders/knees/ankles can't take that kind of exercise, so you're interested in cycling.

➤ You'd consider buying a cycling computer to track mileage.

➤ You want to set distance or time goals and build on them.

➤ Your friends/spouse/child have been egging you on to ride with them, and it looks like fun.

➤ You want to explore the terrain around where you live.

➤ You want to build your mental strength as well as your physical.

➤ You're self-motivated and like to create your own goals.

hill climbing and the bigger challenges. In the meantime, you'll always know that the reward will follow.

The Fitness Bicycle

As with any type of riding, you can get the same ride accomplished on any road bicycle—the ride quality will just differ. Fitness riders are generally looking for a balance between weight, durability, and budget. Of course, those with the biggest budgets can afford the lightest bikes, but those are not necessarily the most reliable. Like any tool used for hours on end, your bike is going to undergo some wear and tear. Although it may be tempting to get the lightest bike, when the parts do wear out (and they will) they'll be much more expensive to replace. Even racers (whom we'll talk about in the next chapter) often have one bike for training and another, lighter bike for race day.

CHAPTER 3

GO! GO! GO!:
The Racing Cyclist

YOU'VE WATCHED THE PROS FROM AFAR AND NOW YOU'RE inspired to test your limits. Fitness riding seems a little too unstructured for your goals. You're ready to pin on your race number and head for the start line.

Why Racing Might Be Calling You

If you're a road racer, it's likely that you already know it. One sure sign: You are already skimming this book for the sections on training, nutrition, and getting a leg up on the competition. Bike racing tends to appeal to the driven, the stubborn, the gutsy, and, of course, the competitive.

There is something very enticing about speed. The wind in your face, the burning lungs, the thrill of pushing corners with just over 2 centimeters of rubber between you and the road—in the sport of cycle racing, that velocity is mostly dependent on your strength, fearlessness, and cunning. How quickly you go up, how much risk you take to be the first one down the hill, how wisely you use the energy of the riders around you—and possibly your team—to conserve energy all make a difference in a race situation.

Road Racing Lingo Cheat Sheet

- **ATTACK:** A surprise move to get ahead of a group of riders
- **BELL LAP:** The final lap of a race
- **BLOCK:** To position yourself in front of or as a team surrounding competing riders to give your teammate an advantage
- **BREAKAWAY:** To successfully attack and ride away from the main pack
- **BOXED IN:** Trapped by a group of riders in a pack, completely blocked on all sides
- **CAT (CATEGORY):** Divisions in competition levels. In the United States it breaks down as follows: Cat 5: Beginner; Cat 4: Novice; Cat 3: Sport; Cat 2: Expert; Cat 1: Elite. Racers must earn a certain number of podium placements or race points before moving ("catting") up to the next category.
- **DRAFT:** To use a rider in front of you to block the wind by riding in their slipstream, making it much easier to maintain speed
- **JUMP OR KICK:** A quick acceleration, sometimes developing into a full attack
- **LEAD OUT:** To help another rider by attacking while that rider drafts your wheel, pulling them out of the peloton to gain a better position for a sprint. This conserves the sprinter's energy to give him or her the edge to win.
- **MASS START:** A race where all the contestants line up at the starting line as a group and take off together at the same time

To become a good racer you'll also have to enjoy structure. From following training plans, to observing strict nutrition and hydration standards, to getting the hours of sleep that are key to repairing muscles to take the next day's beating, road racing can be more than a hobby. Due to the time commitment, it can quickly become both a lifestyle and an identity.

People who are new to cycling but attracted to racing tend to have an athletic background. Runners, skiers, and basketball, football, tennis, and hockey players find themselves looking at two wheels—either to add to their training or as an option after an injury pushes them out of their current sport. Activities that are hard on joints or have a high incidence of injury are creators of racing cyclists. However, you don't need to be an athlete to enjoy the sport. All you really need is a competitive streak.

What Road Racing Looks Like

If you're not convinced this is your forte, be aware there are a variety of types of racing on the road. Regardless of the type of race, you'll be training. This looks similar to fitness riding, but your time on the bike will be much more regimented to optimize your race results. Truth be told, road racing starts not on the

➤ **OVERLAP:** A rider's front wheel overtaking the wheel of the rider he or she is drafting. Extremely dangerous when riding in a pack

➤ **PELOTON OR PACK:** The main group of riders—also called a bunch or field

➤ **POPPED OFF THE BACK:** When a rider loses power and falls out of the peloton, usually getting left behind in the race (also known as "getting dropped")

➤ **PODIUM:** The collective term for first-, second-, and third-place riders who will all stand on a three-tiered stage to receive their prizes (which are the only ones usually awarded)

➤ **PRIMES:** In criterium racing, small prizes that are awarded on certain laps to add excitement and strategy to the race

➤ **PULL:** To go to the front of the peloton where there is little protection from the wind and set or maintain the pace. Generally, throughout the race different riders will take turns pulling because it's the hardest position to ride in.

➤ **SPRINT:** A quick dash for the finish line or other designated competition within the race, like a mountaintop or prime. Sprint winners are not just decided by the fastest person, but by how the riders have positioned themselves both just before and during the attempt.

➤ **WHEEL SUCKING:** To always stay behind someone's draft and never take your turn pulling at the front. Not looked upon kindly, but sometimes a good strategy

bike but by looking at your local or regional race schedule, then deciding which races you want to participate in and if there is one race in particular that you want to "peak" at (or try to win). In this sport, even races are a part of your training for the big performance of the season.

Racing bicycles is not an activity that you'll do from home. After all that time training on the road, you may have to drive significant distances to get to the races. Beyond time, there's also an added financial investment. You'll need to buy an annual state or national racing license and entry fee for each race.

Because it's dictated by a calendar, road racing is both seasonal and cyclical. Depending on the weather where you live, there will be a season that racers rest and recover, a prerace season training, and sometimes a long (more than 6 months) race season.

Types of Road Racing

The beautiful thing about road racing is that there's a little something for everyone. You can dip your toes in with a time trial or go for the whole enchilada with a stage race. All of these take place on paved roads.

CIRCUIT racing is often what most people imagine a road race to be. A mass start that takes place on some kind of large loop—usually from 5 to 25 miles—that competitors cover for a specific number of laps. It is usually a longer distance race (men cover around 60 to 100 miles, women around 40 to 80 miles) that takes place over one day. Riding in the middle of the *peloton,* racers are both protected from wind and pulled along by the speed of the riders surrounding them, giving opportunities to rest and recover after the overall speed of the *pack* surges. In this kind of race, it's extremely helpful to have a team or people you work with to take turns *pulling* to help you stay in the *peloton* without getting *popped off the back.* Teamwork and cunning are key factors since you're trying to conserve energy over a longer period of time. If you like working with others and games with strategy, this type of racing might be for you.

POINT-TO-POINT road races are the brothers of circuit races, with the same kind of race start and similar skills required but with tactical differences. In a circuit race, riders will have a chance to get to know the quirks of the course and their opponents over every lap. During a point-to-point race every moment is new, so it's harder to predict how your competitors might handle changes in terrain and tactics. Also, it's not uncommon for these courses to include steeper, longer climbs.

CRITERIUMS ("CRITS") are as thrilling for spectators as they are for competitors. It's also a mass start race, but the course is a very short—usually 1 mile or less in length—loop.

Instead of curves, visualize lots of turns around tight corners in city blocks. These courses are often the crown jewel of urban areas. The course may follow only a few blocks before screaming around another turn, but the racers are often traveling at speeds well over 20 miles per hour in a *pack* so close together that shoulders touch and handlebars are in danger of hooking, making positioning key and technical bike-handling skills a must. Crits usually last for shorter time periods, but at a much higher overall intensity than circuit racing. *Primes* are offered to make the race more exciting by encouraging different riders to sprint throughout the race instead of conserving energy for the big win at the end. Even if you don't have a chance at the *podium, primes* are a good way to practice *sprinting* within the race.

TIME TRIAL is the only road race that doesn't have a mass start. This time, it's you (or your team riding as a group) against the clock for the fastest overall time. The courses are usually 10 to 25 miles in length, can be flat, hilly, or entirely uphill, and often play to the strengths of endurance riders who can hold a very hard pace steadily for a long time. In triathlons, time trials are the biking portion of the swim-bike-run race. In this racing, there are no *packs* to rest in and no sprints or surges to keep pace with. You are going it alone, and this is a mind over matter style of racing.

STAGE RACES are a combination of some or all the above rolled into one fantastic event.

The most famous example is the Tour de France, which features most of these types of racing, but over a course of nearly 21 days straight. Don't worry, your local races won't be that tough. There will sometimes be multiple races in 1 day or spread out over a series of days. These events favor the "all rounder" rider, someone who is fairly good at all the qualities needed for each type of racing.

What a Road Racer Looks Like

Unlike other road cyclists, road racers share a similar general body type—at least after they've been racing a season or two. Because many races are won or lost during a hill climb, the weight of the racer is as influential as his or her power. An extremely strong racer who is a few pounds overweight is at a significant disadvantage to his or her fellow racer. In road racing, it's very important in most cases to stay with the racing group and not get left behind, and carrying those few extra pounds requires more energy from riders just when they're already riding at their max. This is also why it is critical for racers to concentrate on nutrition both on and off the bike. Some professional racers look almost skeletal during their season, but they have an entire staff of doctors, trainers, and nutritionists checking in on them every day to make sure they're healthy. Anyone can starve themselves thin, but for the average Joe or Jane,

it's almost impossible to lose that much weight and still get the proper vitamins and energy you'll need to sustain training and racing. That being said, it is possible to lose weight with the proper training and diet. Racing alone burns an enormous amount of calories.

Racers are divided by age and skill level, so if you're concerned about where to start, you'll be placed with people who are roughly your age and ability at your first race.

What a Race Bike Looks Like

Typically, you want a racing bike to be a light-weight machine for the same reason the racer's body needs to be carrying as little as possible. In either case, added weight is not an advantage

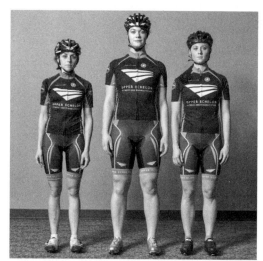

A quick look at a race team shows that different body types play to different strengths—like climbing, sprinting, or endurance.

in racing, so counting your bicycle's pounds—or even grams—can make a difference on the finish line.

Time-trial bicycles are different from the average road bike. Time-trial bikes are very light, mostly meant for riding flat terrain and have a very unique, aerodynamic riding position. This means where and how the rider sits and pedals is different from on other road bikes. It's most recognizable by the bent forward position and armrests that come forward off the handlebars. You can outfit a regular road bike with arm rests to adapt the bike to be time-trial ready, or you can buy a time-trial-specific bike that is built around this special, aerodynamic position.

Regardless of the type of racing, you can hit the start line with any style of road bike. Some riders swap out parts on their bikes—for example, a lighter weight set of wheels and tires—on race day for a little extra advantage without having to own a second road bike.

Top Signs You Might Be a Bike Racer

➤ If you're not pushing yourself, you're not having fun.

➤ You like to compete, but more importantly to win.

➤ You're already racing in another sport or discipline and you want a new challenge.

➤ You don't want to track only mileage, but also power output, heart rate, and any other measure of your fitness on a daily basis.

➤ You eat goals for breakfast.

➤ You'll ride—rain or shine, indoors or out—every day.

➤ Your mental strength is as tough as your physical.

➤ You're willing to hire a coach and have your life on the bike revolve around specific training plans.

➤ You're interested in visiting a place called "The Pain Cave."

Team or Rogue?

As you enter into this sport, you want to decide early in the season if you want to join a team or go it alone. Many beginners spend their first season as free agents (a term that makes it seem more glamorous than it actually is). Starting off "unattached" gives you a chance to get your legs underneath you and start to understand the rhythms of how the races ebb and flow, and gives you a great appreciation of how racing

works. It's also a great way to watch how other teams work and "get to know" them. Each will have its own vibe, which will depend on who is on it, who's in charge, and how organized they are. Some teams are more social, some more competitive, some both.

If you're going to race time trials exclusively, the only benefit to being on a team is that you'll have other people to train with, maybe drive with to the races, and decompress with after the races are over. Since the time trial is focused on the individual, teams aren't of much help on the course.

For circuit, crit, point-to-point, and especially stage races, having a team is a big advantage. Staying in the peloton of the race is a huge plus because it conserves energy, and it's easier to stay in the main field if your team has its own mini-pack to help keep one another there. Your team can also shield you from other riders' tactics or set you up for a winning sprint.

Of course, if you're riding as part of a team, it might be your position in a race to help another team rider to do the same.

Being part of a team can be helpful in training, too. Having more knowledgeable riders to show you the ropes in training and practice race scenarios is invaluable. Fellow racers can have valuable intel on training techniques and the latest gadgets, and can foster a sense of community and support that is pure gold on days when you don't make the podium.

PART II

THE BIKE IS THE SUM OF ITS PARTS

Bikes seem simple . . . until you arrive at the shop and the salesperson seems to be speaking French. Maybe this is because until now biking has been as easy as getting on and riding—which you've been doing since you were a kid—so you feel like you should know this stuff. And you find yourself reluctant to mention that you barely passed Spanish in high school, so you don't have the faintest clue what they're talking about.

Don't despair. Think of this section as a simple and common "phrase book" you might take when journeying to a foreign country (a.k.a. your local bike shop) to learn important phrases and customs—so you're not completely lost and can figure out how to find the bathroom and other important things you'll want to know.

Hopefully by now you have a good idea of what type of riding you might want to start doing, and maybe you have opened your mind to the possibilities of how far your bike really can take you. Now it's time to prep for your bike-buying journey.

We'll start by breaking down how a bike is put together, so you have a better idea of what parts are on the bike, what their quality is, and how that reflects how much they cost. Then you'll get the intel on your actual bike-buying journey and what to expect. You want the best deal possible for the closest match to your needs, and this will help you find it. After you buy the bike, you might think you're ready to roll. You mostly are—except for a few add-ons and upgrades, some which are common choices (like what pedals to buy) and some that you may just want to have to make your riding experience better.

Ready to do some learning? Class is officially in session.

CHAPTER 4

The Geography of a Road Bike

The Suspension System

As we now know, the *frame* and *fork* are the main parts of the bicycle that the bike company makes. The frame consists of four main tubes and two sets of smaller tubes that make up two triangles.

The *top*, *seat*, *head*, and *down tubes* make up the front triangle. The stiffness of these tubes makes your bike stable and helps support the weight of your body. The seat tube stiffness is very important as it can influence how much power transfers from your body to the pedals. The rear wheel sits inside the back triangle and is made up of the *seat stays* (that connect near the seat), *chain stays* that follow the run of your chain, and, again, the *seat tube*. The two triangles are put together at the factory, then the rest of the parts are added to it.

The *fork*, which looks like a musical tuning fork, is separate from the frame but is designed by the manufacturer to work specifically with the frame. Some forks can be swapped out for aftermarket upgrades, but it's pretty unusual if you're buying a bike directly from a shop.

All these parts make up what is commonly considered the "frame" but sometimes referred to as the "frame and fork." By changing the angles of these triangles and of

(continued on page 28)

Diagram of a Road Bicycle

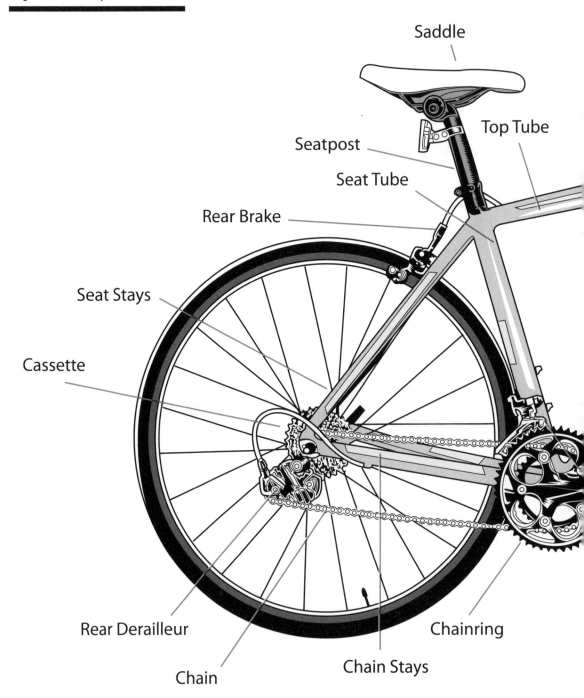

Saddle

Seatpost

Seat Tube

Rear Brake

Top Tube

Seat Stays

Cassette

Rear Derailleur

Chain

Chain Stays

Chainring

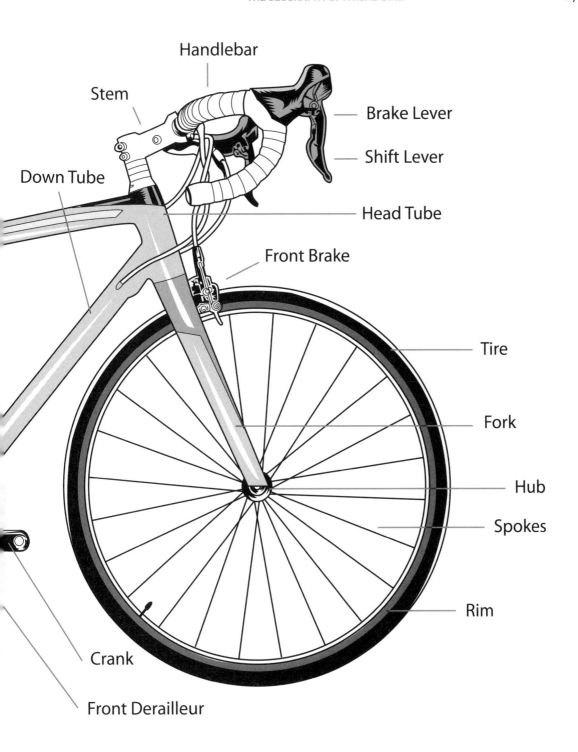

Handlebar

Stem

Brake Lever

Shift Lever

Down Tube

Head Tube

Front Brake

Tire

Fork

Hub

Spokes

Rim

Crank

Front Derailleur

the fork (as well as the material they're built with), manufacturers can manipulate how the ride feels when you're on the bike.

Most people are familiar with *wheels,* but don't understand that they actually consist of three main parts: the *rim,* the *spokes,* and the *hub* (the center of the wheel that spins). It's important to appreciate what wheels do for the quality of your time on the road. They are both your support system and suspension, which makes them one of the hardest working parts of your bike. The type of wheels you want will vary greatly depending on your riding style. Inertia makes them heavier, so rims and tires take more energy to get moving. In the case of racing, a lighter wheel can give a huge advantage. For commuting or touring, you'll want a nice, heavy rim and stout tire to support the extra weight you'll be carrying and to prevent flats. Wheels are the most expensive components on the bike after the frame and fork— sometimes even more expensive in the case of ultralight race sets. All that being said, it's likely you'll just stick with the wheels that come with the bike you buy, as they'll be designed to work best with it.

The *quick release (or QR) skewers* are what fasten your wheels to the frame. They were designed to make it easy to get the wheel on and off—for storing or transporting the bike or for changing a flat. They're simple to use—once you know how to use them correctly. If you're not absolutely sure you know how they work, the bike shop will be happy to take a few minutes to show you; then go home and practice a few times so you cement it in your brain. If you use them incorrectly, you can damage your hub (making it much harder to pedal) or your wheel can come loose while riding.

Tires come with the package when you buy the bike, and their width, durability, and ride quality vary as much as wheels. The width of the tire is directly connected to its use. Narrower tires are usually found on racing or fitness bikes and wider tires on commuter or touring bikes. Basically, heavier tires are just like the heavier wheels: They'll be sturdier and less likely to go flat, but slower and harder to get rolling. Tires are the component most likely to be skimped on when bike manufacturers are putting together the complete package, so it's likely it's something you might upgrade right after you get your bike.

Tubes are found inside the tires and are what actually hold the air to make the tire fill up. Tubes are mainly made in one big factory in Taiwan, so their quality is fairly comparable across the board. For road bikes, the valve stems (where you put the air in) are usually Presta valves. These valves look skinny and have a tiny nubbin at the top that can be unscrewed to let air in or out. If you've never used them, ask your shop for a quick lesson before you walk out the door.

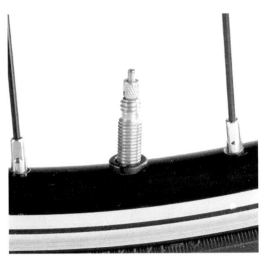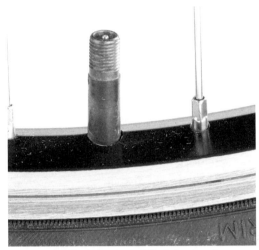

On the left is the skinnier Presta valve, usually found on road bikes. On the right is the larger, chubbier Schrader valve.

Your *saddle* (also called a *seat*) helps cushion the road and supports your body weight so you can transition power to the pedals. Though a bigger saddle seems better (especially when you're just starting out and you'll have more soreness), there are great reasons road saddles are the shape and size they are. Many, many riders swap out saddles from what comes stock with the bike, so we'll discuss more about this in both Chapter 11, Upgrades and Add-Ons, and Part IV, The Fit.

Beneath your saddle is the *seatpost,* which attaches the saddle to the frame and is adjustable for height. This makes it so a generic bike size can be somewhat tailored to your body.

Under your hands reside the *handlebars.* Their depth and width adjust with the frame size, so a smaller frame will have narrower,

shallower bars than a larger one. This is the key to a comfortable ride. There are three main hand positions on the handlebars, and this variability is what gives them their shape and saves you from sleepy or painful hands. The most common is resting your hands on top of the levers (called the hoods) where your fingers can easily reach both the brakes and shifters. When you're cruising along or want to sit up a bit, you'll use the top, flat part of the bars that are horizontal to the rider. The U-shaped curved parts of the bars are commonly referred to as the *drops.* The lowest part is the best place for you to descend because it helps lower your center of gravity. The handlebars not only support you, but in conjunction with the *bar tape* wrapped around them, they cushion your upper body from fatiguing road vibration.

Stop and Go

There are only two things you really need the bike to do: go, and, of course, stop. These two simple ideas are accomplished with the use of the brakes, shifting, and drivetrain (which means the part you push to propel forward).

Integrated shifters are the most common style on road bikes. As the name "integrated" implies, they combine two things—the shift lever and the brake lever—into one lever. The shift function helps you change gears (making it easier or harder to pedal) and the break function is what you pull on to stop. Both have cables that connect them to the parts they need to control. On a road bike, you'll usually ride on the *hoods* of the levers (the rubbery, horn-shaped part that extends out from the top of the handlebar) because that's where you have the most control over shifting and braking, as well as the best balance.

The *brakes* (or *brake calipers*) are just above

The Great Chainring Divides

WHEN CHOOSING A BIKE, ONE OF THE main questions you'll be faced with is "Do you want a *standard double,* a *triple,* or a *compact double*?" This is not about espresso or liqueur shots (though you might wish it was). They're asking how many chainrings—the gears in the front on your crank arm—you want. How many you have and how you choose will greatly affect the experience you have when riding, particularly when climbing. Even on the same make and model of one bike, you may be offered a choice of which style you want, so it's important to understand how they differ so you can choose the best fit for you.

The number of teeth (the little notches on the chainring) determines how hard it is to pedal in that gear. The more teeth, the bigger the circle, the harder it is to make the bike move. Most bikes come with at least a big gear and a small gear. You use the larger, higher-tooth-count gear for flats and going downhill, and a smaller one with fewer teeth to help you get up hills.

For a long time your only two choices were what is now called a *standard double* and a *triple.* The standard double has two rings that are both fairly big. Years ago it was your only choice on most road bikes built for racing or fitness. The problem was that if you lived somewhere that had large hills and you weren't a strong climber, getting up them was a struggle.

To help with this, you sometimes had a choice to buy a bike that came with a *triple,* or a three-geared chainring. This was good because it gave you a variety of choices, the smallest making hill climbing accessible and easy, the middle being what you rode in most of the time, and the large for going down hills or picking up momentum on the down slope of a dip. The bad news was that this third ring added quite a bit of weight. It wasn't a problem for touring bikes (on which you're carrying a heavy load so triples are always installed because without them it's nearly impossible to climb) but on race bikes, many people wanted to save the weight, so they simply suffered on climbs.

your wheels and have rubber pads that clamp down on the rim of the wheel when you pull the brake lever, making you stop. Your lever should neither pull the lever all the way to the handlebar nor be set so hard to grab that it hurts your hand to hold it down for more than a few moments. In either case, you want to have good control over the brake lever.

The "drivetrain" is a fancy name for all the components that work together to make your bike move forward. It consists of the *chain*, *crank arms*, *chainrings* (a.k.a. front gears), *cassette* (a.k.a. rear gears), and *front* and *rear derailleurs*. Don't let all those fancy, foreign terms overwhelm you. Just know that they all work together and on new bikes are all usually sold together as a package from one component manufacturer. They're easily identifiable by being the dirtiest, greasiest parts on your bike, because they need lubrication to do their jobs. When you oil your chain, it spreads to the rest of the drivetrain, allowing the components to play

In this century, science came out proving that faster pedaling (called cadence) was more efficient, saved your energy, and made you a better rider. So there became a market for smaller, easier gears on a fitness or a racing bike. This is when the *compact double* made its debut, changing the world of fitness and racing cycling forever. It comes with a small gear that is slightly bigger than the lowest gear in a triple but much smaller than the standard double, and a big gear that is slightly smaller than the biggest gear on a triple or a standard double. This makes it so the gear sizes are close enough that the chain could still shift smoothly from one to the other.

Let's talk turkey. If you're riding a touring bike, there's no debate. You want it to come with a *triple*. Anything else won't offer gears that are easy enough to carry the load uphill.

For a fitness or recreational rider, there's a lot more contention. If you're not a very strong climber and you live, for example, in the mountains or foothills, you'll likely want to invest in a compact double. It really offers the best of both worlds. But if you want the easiest gear possible and don't mind the extra weight, you can still get your fitness/recreational/racing bike with a triple.

If it's flat as a pancake where you live (meaning there's no hill that's longer than a quarter mile), you'll likely be just as happy with a standard double. This is often what racers prefer. However, even in these areas some riders like the idea of being able to have the more versatile gearing that a compact double offers.

Before you buy, be sure to test ride bikes that will work for your terrain, fitness, and riding style, and don't let the salesperson talk you out of what you have decided you like after test riding. Their riding style or fitness might be quite different from yours.

nicely together, keeping quiet and smooth on the road.

Although the *pedals* aren't officially part of the drivetrain, they attach to the crank arms and give you the platform to push on to make the drivetrain move. We'll talk more about the different pedal choices you might want on your bike in Chapter 11. Many road bikes are not sold with pedals because riders develop individual preferences for specific brands, so if anything, the bike sometimes comes with a "test ride" pedal that is cheap and expendable.

And the Wheels Go Round and Round

Anything on your bike that spins or turns has to have *bearings* inside to keep it rolling freely. In the case of your bike, these are located inside your *hubs, pedals,* and head tube (called *headset bearings,* which allow you to steer) and near your crank arms (called the *bottom bracket,* which allows your crank arms to turn and makes pedaling easy). When shopping for your first road bike, these parts are the least important to your purchase.

CHAPTER 5

Component Breakdown

BICYCLES ARE A COMPILATION OF ABOUT 25 TO 30 DIFFERENT parts (usually referred to as *components*), designed and manufactured by just as many different parts brands, that have been bolted onto a frame and fork to make a complete bike. The frame and fork are always designed by bicycle companies. You might have even heard of a few—Trek, Giant, Specialized, Cannondale, and Ridley are some of the more well-known brands. So as a buyer, you may think that if you're familiar with the bike brand, you should be able to walk in and buy a great bike.

However, there are all those other little parts we've just described (such as wheels, brakes, cranks, and handlebars) that attach to the frame and fork to create a complete bicycle. When you're shopping for, say, a blender or a car, you don't need to

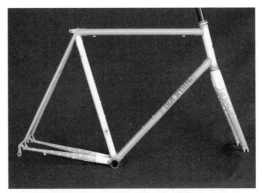

When you think of a bike "brand" you don't always realize that this is all they make—all the other parts are added on from different companies.

do too much research into who made the side panel or gears in the motor. Unfortunately, this doesn't really apply to bikes.

A single frame manufacturer buys all the smaller parts from many different suppliers. These are all the little pieces that come together on and in the frame to make a bicycle as you know it, and all of these parts are interchangeable between manufacturers. After frame assembly, one complete bike can be outfitted from a few different suppliers. Each comes with its own reputation, and slight performance differences affect the bike and how it interacts with your body.

To keep costs down, a bicycle company will make a deal with a few different component manufacturers to purchase the parts in bulk for an entire bike line. If you bought these parts individually, it would cost much more than buying them bundled together on a complete bike. It's important to know a bit about not only which of those parts you might be asked about by the salesperson, but also who the main suppliers of those components are, the basic comparisons of how they work, and how price affects quality.

Most important of those, the quality of your components is directly related to the price of your bike. Wondering what the difference really is between the $1,200 bike and the $2,300 bike? The frames might be very similar, but the more expensive option will likely come equipped with components that are more durable, lighter,

and higher quality, meaning they'll both perform better and last longer.

Think of two examples we all use every day: electronics and kitchen knives. With electronics—like your computer or smart phone—the speed and capability (and, in some cases, durability, too) of the machine increases with cost. With kitchen knives, the more it costs, the longer it will stay sharp, the easier it is to maintain, and the less likelihood of accidentally drawing blood. A high-quality knife can last lifetimes if it's well taken care of—which is why we'll be looking into how to care for all these components in Part X, Tuning Your Ride.

What the Heck is a Grouppo (and Why Do I Care)?

Out of all the words that get thrown around in bike shops, *grouppo* (the Italian word for "group") smacks particularly of the kind of snobbery that people associate with bike shops. It's really just a fancy word for a single collection of components from one manufacturer, also called a group set or, even more clearly, a component package. These include the shift/brake levers, chain, cassette, crankset, bottom bracket, and brake calipers, and as mentioned before, they are often sold in bulk as a package deal to bicycle manufacturers from component manufacturers to keep costs down.

Making things a little more complicated, each of the major component manufacturers has

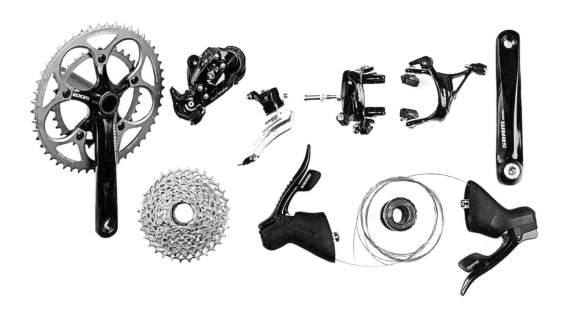

There are a lot of little parts in a group set that make your bike complete.

multiple tiers of these collections that you might be offered on any given bike. There are three to five levels for each manufacturer, but the one thing that all of them have in common is that as the price increases so does the quality, while at the same time they get lighter.

It's good to get acquainted with the styles and terms because when you start looking at bicycles, their main differences are going to be in three areas: frame materials (which we'll discuss in Chapter 7), wheel sets (which we'll discuss in Chapter 11), and what group set they come outfitted with.

No matter what style of riding you'll be doing,

these options will remain fairly consistent across the board on both new and used bikes.

The Names You'll See When You Shop: Shimano, SRAM, and Campagnolo

Shimano

This is the largest supplier of bicycle components in North America, though their home base is Japan. (You'll be surprised to learn that their other biggest seller is . . . fishing reels. Surprising, but true.)

Shimano has gotten to be a market leader because of its solid product and great reputation since 1961. Since then, it has developed its road component line (it also has mountain and city bike lines) into two tiers of quality, with smaller levels within each division. This system offers buyers a variety of choices. Shimano has something in just about every budget and quality level. This is one indicator of how much the sport of road cycling has grown in the past 40 years, because the market now has a need for a lot of options.

SRAM

This U.S. company until recently was mostly known for its dependable mountain bike and city bike components. If you have ever ridden a bike with "twist" style shifters, they were likely made by SRAM. After breaking into Shimano's market share in the early 1990s, SRAM grew its mountain and commuter component lines and solidified their place in the cycling market.

In 2006 SRAM introduced its first line of road components. Since then it has developed its own market niche by concentrating mainly on the highest level of components but also offering a new system that is specifically made to help people climb more easily. SRAM's additions to the road market in the past few years have really helped push all the major competitors to innovate.

Campagnolo

This Italian company (often referred to as "Campy" for short) is the oldest and has a stellar reputation. It was founded in 1933 and has not since wavered from a dedication to road components. Campagnolo is famous for breaking new ground and innovating—in fact, it was the first to successfully create reliable rear derailleurs. This is the only major manufacturer that does not offer mountain or city bike parts, because it is committed to creating the best possible experience with road bicycles. Campagnolo's prices also reflect this commitment to quality.

For many years (before SRAM entered the arena), Campagnolo was Shimano's main competitor. Like Shimano, it offers two tiers of components with smaller divisions between them, as well as components that are outside the traditional group set, such as wheels and seatposts.

How Their Stuff Works

One of the most important aspects of what parts your bike comes with is how they function and feel in your hands and on the road. For all three companies, the brakes and gears work almost exactly the same. The big differences are in how each lever makes its shift and how large the grip is on the lever.

Shimano

Shimano is known for its medium-sized brake/shifter levers that fit medium to large hands well (the exception being its electronic shifting, which has much smaller levers and works well for smaller hands as well). Its shifter is built into the same lever as the brake and moves easily and quietly, which is nice for hands that aren't as strong but which may not be preferred if you're someone who likes to feel each shift click decisively.

SRAM

The SRAM shifter is the largest—meaning it takes more of your hand to wrap around it and to get a grip. Like Shimano, SRAM's shifter is also built into the brake lever (in a slightly different way, however, because of patents), fits large to medium hands well, and has a very firm and exact shifting click. This means it takes more leverage to move it, which also makes having strong hands a plus.

Campagnolo

This shifting system is the most elegant, with the smallest hood (both in length and in how small the handgrip is), making it ideal for smaller hands. Campy gives a firm click of chain moving to a different gear (like SRAM) but with easy shifting (like Shimano). This lever also moves part of the shifting away from the brake lever to a small tab for your thumb to shift in one direction—this gives you better leverage. This tab also helps make the whole lever smaller in size.

What Their Stuff Costs

Again, since the bicycle companies buy the parts in bulk, we'll break down the cost of the bike that you'll see the parts on, instead of the cost of the parts themselves. Occasionally bicycle manufacturers will mix and match a part or two from a more inexpensive group to help lower the overall cost of the bike, so just because the shifters are at one price point doesn't mean the derailleur isn't a more inexpensive one.

The bottom line is that if you plan on riding 1,000 miles or more a year (which sounds like a lot until you realize that can be as few as two 20-mile rides a week over 6 months), you can easily wear through the parts of a sub-$2,000 bike in 2 to 3 years. Often the replacement parts on these bikes are half the cost of a new bike. It can pay off later to spend a little more now on the entry level of upper tier components that will last 7 to 10 years.

(See the handy chart on the next page to keep all the names, prices, and comparisons straight.)

Shimano

Shimano has the widest range of price points and so is best suited to work with any budget.

(continued on page 40)

Group Sets

SHIMANO COMPONENTS

➤ DURA ACE DI2 (ELECTRIC)	➤ DURA ACE	➤ ULTEGRA DI2 (ELECTRIC)	➤ ULTEGRA
Performance: Highest	**Performance:** Excellent	**Performance:** Excellent	**Performance:** Very good
Durability: Excellent	**Durability:** Excellent	**Durability:** Excellent	**Durability:** Very good
Materials: Ultra lightweight, high-tech	**Materials:** Ultra lightweight, high-tech	**Materials:** Ultra lightweight, high-tech	**Materials:** Very lightweight
Replacement Parts Available: No	**Replacement Parts Available:** No	**Replacement Parts Available:** No	**Replacement Parts Available:** No
Lever Size: Small	**Lever Size:** Medium to large	**Lever Size:** Small	**Lever Size:** Medium to large
Shift Feel: Definitive, crisp (with cool electronic noise)	**Shift Feel:** Soft, very smooth	**Shift Feel:** Definitive (with electronic noise)	**Shift Feel:** Soft, smooth
Difficulty of Shift: Effortless (push button)	**Difficulty of Shift:** Light touch	**Difficulty of Shift:** Effortless (push button)	**Difficulty of Shift:** Light touch
Cost: Stock on bikes costing $5,000+	**Cost:** Stock on bikes costing $3,200+	**Cost:** Stock on bikes costing $3,200+	**Cost:** Stock on bikes costing $1,800+

➤ 105	➤ TIAGRA	➤ SORA
Performance: Good, dependable	**Performance:** Fair	**Performance:** Fair to poor
Durability: Very good	**Durability:** Fair	**Durability:** Fair to poor
Materials: Somewhat lightweight	**Materials:** Not lightweight	**Materials:** Heaviest
Replacement Parts Available: No	**Replacement Parts Available:** No	**Replacement Parts Available:** No
Lever Size: Medium to large	**Lever Size:** Medium to large	**Lever Size:** Medium to large
Shift Feel: Soft	**Shift Feel:** Soft, some resistance	**Shift Feel:** Soft with resistance
Difficulty of Shift: Light to medium touch	**Difficulty of Shift:** Easy	**Difficulty of Shift:** Easy
Cost: Stock on bikes costing $1,500+	**Cost:** Stock on bikes costing $900+	**Cost:** Stock on bikes costing $700+

SRAM COMPONENTS

➤ RED	➤ RIVAL	➤ FORCE
Performance: Excellent	**Performance:** Very good	**Performance:** Good
Durability: Highest	**Durability:** Very good	**Durability:** Good
Materials: Ultra lightweight, high-tech	**Materials:** Very light, high-tech	**Materials:** Light, high-tech
Replacement Parts Available: No	**Replacement Parts Available:** No	**Replacement Parts Available:** No
Lever Size: Medium to large	**Lever Size:** Medium to large	**Lever Size:** Medium to large
Shift Feel: Exact, crisp, definitive	**Shift Feel:** Crisp, definitive	**Shift Feel:** Crisp
Difficulty of Shift: Hard/firm	**Difficulty of Shift:** Hard/firm	**Difficulty of Shift:** Hard/firm
Cost: On bikes costing $3,000+	**Cost:** Stock on bikes costing $2,500+	**Cost:** Stock on bikes costing $1,750+

CAMPAGNOLO COMPONENTS

➤ SUPER RECORD EPS (ELECTRONIC SHIFTING)	➤ SUPER RECORD	➤ RECORD EPS (ELECTRONIC SHIFTING)
Performance: Excellent	**Performance:** Excellent	**Performance:** Excellent
Durability: Excellent	**Durability:** Excellent	**Durability:** Excellent
Materials: Lightweight, high-tech	**Materials:** Ultra lightweight, high-tech	**Materials:** Ultra lightweight, high-tech
Replacement Parts Available: Yes	**Replacement Parts Available:** Yes	**Replacement Parts Available:** Yes
Lever Size: Small/Compact	**Lever Size:** Small/Compact	**Lever Size:** Small/Compact
Shift Feel: Definitive, crisp (with cool electronic noise)	**Shift Feel:** Crisp, clean	**Shift Feel:** Definitive, crisp (with cool electronic noise)
Difficulty of Shift: Effortless (push button)	**Difficulty of Shift:** Very easy	**Difficulty of Shift:** Effortless (push button)
Cost: On bikes costing $11,000+	**Cost:** Stock on bikes costing $9,000+	**Cost:** Stock on bikes costing $9,000+

➤ RECORD	➤ CHORUS	➤ ATHENA EPS (ELECTRONIC SHIFTING)
Performance: Excellent	**Performance:** Very, very good	**Performance:** Excellent
Durability: Very, very good	**Durability:** Very good	**Durability:** Very good
Materials: Very lightweight, high-tech	**Materials:** Lightweight	**Materials:** Heavy
Replacement Parts Available: Yes	**Replacement Parts Available:** Yes	**Replacement Parts Available:** Yes
Lever Size: Small/Compact	**Lever Size:** Small/Compact	**Lever Size:** Small/Compact
Shift Feel: Crisp, clean	**Shift Feel:** Crisp, clean	**Shift Feel:** Definitive, crisp (with cool electronic noise)
Difficulty of Shift: Easy	**Difficulty of Shift:** Easy	**Difficulty of Shift:** Effortless (push button)
Cost: Stock on bikes costing $6,500+	**Cost:** Stock on bikes costing $5,000+	**Cost:** Stock on bikes costing $6,500+

➤ ATHENA	➤ CENTAUR	➤ VELOCE
Performance: Good	**Performance:** Good	**Performance:** Fair
Durability: Very good	**Durability:** Good	**Durability:** Good
Materials: Average	**Materials:** Heavy	**Materials:** Heavy
Replacement Parts Available: Yes	**Replacement Parts Available:** Yes	**Replacement Parts Available:** Yes
Lever Size: Small/Compact	**Lever Size:** Small/Compact	**Lever Size:** Small/Compact
Shift Feel: Crisp	**Shift Feel:** Exact	**Shift Feel:** Exact
Difficulty of Shift: Medium	**Difficulty of Shift:** Medium/Firm	**Difficulty of Shift:** Medium/Firm
Cost: Stock on bikes costing $3,500	**Cost:** Stock on bikes costing $3,000+	**Cost:** Stock on bikes costing $2,700+

There are two tiers of components, each with three levels. The top tier brands (Dura Ace, Ultegra, and 105) are built to be the lightest, best performing, and most durable of Shimano's offerings. They are typically found on bikes priced at $2,000 and upward.

This upper tier's finest components are in the Dura Ace series, which is developed for professional racers. The technology and innovations trickle down into the cheaper Ultegra, which is a little heavier and not quite as smooth or durable as Dura Ace, and then to the even less expensive 105, which is heavier again, less smooth, and slightly less durable than either of the others.

The lower tier (Tiagra and Sora) is offered to provide options for those on a budget, but sacrifices weight, performance, durability, and modern upgrades. They are most often found on bicycles that cost less than $2,000. Tiagra is slightly nicer than Sora, but only nominally.

The brand also offers a line called Di2 at the Dura Ace and Ultegra levels that gets rid of cables and uses a battery to power electronic shifting. This technology makes it so that instead of having to move anything mechanically, you make it work with the push of a soft button, making shifting very, very easy and almost flawless compared to anything with cables. This is the most expensive line Shimano offers and out of budget for most entry-level cyclists. These group sets will typically be found only on bikes costing $3,000 and up.

SRAM

SRAM offers only one level of components that is comparable to Shimano's upper tier, meaning you'll find them on bicycles starting around $2,000 and up. These include its Red, Rival, and Force products.

As a group set, these parts cost a few hundred less than Shimano's while their performance and durability are mostly equal. That makes SRAM the most affordable of the three component manufacturers.

Campagnolo (Campy)

Campagnolo, on the other hand, is the most expensive of all the manufacturers. This is for two reasons. One, all of its products are made in Italy, so there are import taxes that raise the price considerably, making Campy much more affordable in Europe. The other reason is that out of all three manufacturers, it is the only one to design its parts so that they are repairable. If a shifter breaks, you don't have to buy an entire new shifter. On the other hand, you have to pay the cost of the replacement parts and labor, and Campy's components wear out more quickly than Shimano's or SRAM's.

Like Shimano, Campangolo has two tiers. The upper tier consists of Super Record, Record, and Chorus. These top-of-the-line products also have a similar trickle-down effect with technology, where the most expensive Record is for racers, and its technology trickles down into the more affordable Chorus, and then Athena. The upper-tier products are also made of the nicest, most lightweight materials.

Campagnolo offers electronic shifting at its Super Record, Record, and more affordable Athena levels. If budget is a consideration for you, this tier might be a little out of your price range—it's typically found on bikes starting around $4,000 and up to $13,000 or more.

Campagnolo's Athena, Centaur, and Veloce make up the lower tier and are comparable to Shimano's or SRAM's lowest level of their top tiers in cost but are not as nice in performance. For some this means if cost is a factor, you might get more bang for your buck with SRAM or Shimano.

PART III

BIKE BUYING GUIDE: FINDING YOUR SOUL MATE

Now that you know what your goals are, it's time to find the bike that will help you reach them. Lucky for you, as with love, there are a lot of fish in the sea. But between makes, models, and shops, bicycle-buying can get overwhelming quickly, sometimes leading you to spin your wheels—and not get started at all.

So don't be shy. Ask around to see if you have any friends who ride and can make recommendations. You should generally know what you're looking for in a bike and remember a test ride is like the "first date." You can always bow out with a "It's not you, it's me" and move on to the next bike.

You can't have it all (but you can get a lot). Sadly, as in all relationships, there will be compromises. Color is important to most first-time buyers—but it is also the most likely option to be thrown out the window after you see what's available in your size and budget. You might want to ride outdoors year-round in the rain but opt for an ultralight road bike that doesn't take full fenders. You could be absolutely certain you want a steel bike, until you test-ride a carbon one. Focus on what fits your body, your budget, and your riding needs, and it won't matter what color or wheel spoke count is beneath you. You'll be too busy enjoying the lovely ride as the miles speed by.

CHAPTER 6

Your Shopping Pop Quiz

NO PRESSURE: THIS IS AN OPEN BOOK TEST, AND THERE ARE NO wrong answers. These questions can help simplify your options, so you don't end up paralyzed with the thousands of choices available to you.

WHERE DO YOU WANT TO RIDE? Depending on your goals, you may be aiming for the bike paths and quiet country roads or into the peloton of your first race. This can affect positioning, materials, and the number and types of gears you'll want. (See Part I, Finding the Right Ride for You, for more on this.)

WHAT KIND OF POSITION ARE YOU MOST COMFORTABLE SITTING IN? Depending on your body's limitations (proportion, previous injuries, etc.) certain bikes may keep you from experiencing pain while riding. For example, riders with back injuries sometimes gravitate to recumbents or more upright road bikes.

HOW FAR AND FAST DO YOU WANT TO GO? Road bikes vary greatly, and today the industry offers bikes that specialize in long endurance hours in the saddle and others that are made for sprinting, climbing, and descending fast.

WHAT ARE MY GOALS? How much you ride now and how much you hope to ride in the future can change. Be sure to buy a bike that can grow with any of your fitness goals.

Wait. That costs HOW much?

IF THIS WILL BE YOUR FIRST ROAD BIKE, welcome to a dreamy experience. Also know that the cost of a road bike can bring new meaning to the words "sticker shock." New, quality road bikes start at about $1,000. A very good quality, lightweight road racer can range between $2,500 and $4,000.

Yep, you read that right. And that's not even anywhere near the cost of really high-end bikes.

It's possible get a new road bike for less than $1,000, but even with minimal mileage it is likely to need expensive new parts in 2 to 3 years that can cost more than half of what you paid for the bike. Investing a little more from the jump will save you money in the long haul. (See a good breakdown of parts and their cost in Chapter 5, Component Breakdown)

Shopping is a balance. You might compromise on a cheaper frame material because the components that the bike is stocked with are a better quality and will last you longer.

WHAT KIND OF WEATHER DO I WANT TO RIDE IN? Many road bikes are not able to fit full fenders or accommodate wider tires that can offer better traction if you plan to ride outdoors year-round and live in a region with inclement weather.

WHAT DO I WANT TO BE ABLE TO CARRY? There's a huge difference between the ultra-light road machine and the hefty touring bike that is built to carry your entire life for weeks on end.

WHAT KIND OF FRAME MATERIAL DO I WANT? If you don't know a lick about frame material, don't fret—we'll break it down in the next chapter. Often what you'll end up with will primarily be dictated by cost, but also by what kind of riding you want to do.

WHAT'S MY BUDGET? Do some research online or in stores to get an idea of the price range of the type of bike you'd like. It helps with the sticker shock that often accompanies road bicycles. It's common to want to keep to a strict number, but buying a bike is similar to investing in fine kitchen knives or computers. The mid-range value will usually last you significantly longer than the cheapest option, so the money you spend today can save you from needing an expensive new bike upgrade in a few years.

CHAPTER 7

Frame Material Shootout

THIS IS A SHORT GUIDE, INTENDED TO GIVE YOU A QUICK RUN-down of how frame materials affect the bike. To clarify, this covers only the frame. All the other components on your bike are usually a combination of these materials.

If you want to get into the nitty-gritty, try searching for "bicycle frame material comparison" on the Internet. Unless you're an engineer who enjoys wildly varying opinions, you'll soon be lost in the minutiae of data. We'll keep it simple for you.

Frame materials are important because they each have very different qualities. Remember in Part I when we asked you what kind of riding you want to do? Maybe you've decided you want a lightweight race bike. Sometimes the lightest weight carbon bike has less durability than a slightly heavier one. There will be trade-offs with any of the materials, so factor that in.

There is also a cost factor. You get what you pay for, so the smaller your budget, the more you sacrifice weight, quality, or both. The highest end of any of these materials is going to have better durability and ride quality, so if you're not sure what material is for you, the best way to feel the difference is to test-ride.

COST is usually a top factor in your investment, but materials have a range of cost within them. For the most part, you're getting what you pay for. If the price seems

(continued on page 48)

Frame Materials

ALUMINUM

This is the most common material, especially at the entry-level price range of lightweight race and fitness bikes. Because of its stiffness, aluminum has good handling and can accelerate well during sprints and climbs. However, aluminum does not absorb shock well, and the number one complaint is that road chatter wears the rider down—making it the least comfortable material to ride.

It's common for manufacturers to use a carbon-aluminum hybrid to help absorb a little shock. Many modern aluminum road bikes come with a carbon fork to help smooth out the ride quality and buffer road vibration into your hands.

COST: Inexpensive

DURABILITY:
➤ Doesn't rust
➤ Highly resistant to failure from dings or falls
➤ In old age, higher rate of frame failure
➤ Not easily repaired

RIDE QUALITY:
➤ Responsive to power output
➤ Harsher road feel can tire out rider

STIFFNESS: High

WEIGHT: Lightweight (depending on the quality of alloy)

GOOD FOR:
➤ Entry-level recreational or fitness riders who want an inexpensive but somewhat lightweight bike
➤ Riders who need a bike for inclement weather

CARBON FIBER

Carbon fiber is one of the most fascinating materials of modern times. Layers of carbon fiber cloth are epoxied (glued) together. Depending on the number of layers, shape, and width of tubing, and pattern and position of the fabric weave, the frame can be very stiff in one direction to give more responsiveness and compliant in another to smooth out road vibration.

Quality carbon is very durable, but some manufacturers sacrifice quality for fewer layers of fabric and epoxy, which creates an extremely lightweight frame that is also easily broken. As with other materials, the cost is usually in direct proportion to the quality.

COST: Expensive

DURABILITY:
➤ Doesn't rust
➤ Very, very strong
➤ Not as resistant to scratches
➤ Easily repaired (but may require shipping to a facility that can repair it)

RIDE QUALITY:
➤ Responsive to power output
➤ Smooth under vibration
➤ Feels like the rider is "floating," because the road vibration is so deadened

STIFFNESS: High (depending on weave)

WEIGHT: Lightweight (depending on the quality of alloy)

BEST FOR:
➤ Riders under 200 pounds who want a lightweight racing or fitness machine and have a budget over $2,000
➤ Touring, long-distance, and all-rounder road bikes are beginning to be made in carbon, but these are in their infancy.

STEEL

Bikes have been made of steel since their inception, making them a classic choice. Because of this, many die-hard fans will claim that "only steel is real" and that other frame materials are inferior.

Although it is tried and true and the newest steel alloys are lighter than ever, it has pros and cons just as any other material. Frames flex a small amount under load. This elasticity gives the rider a lively or springy road feel and can absorb road vibration and bumps, but also sucks away the power transferred to the pedals. This being said, a very high-quality steel frame is the stiffest after carbon fiber.

COST: Inexpensive to high range (varies widely with quality and weight). Lighter, stiffer alloys are more expensive.

DURABILITY:
➤ Very durable
➤ Easily repaired
➤ Prone to rust

RIDE QUALITY:
➤ Smooth and springy
➤ Gives feedback from the road, making your bike gently spring back from bumps and adding to the rider's awareness of small changes in riding surface
➤ Less responsive (the elasticity absorbs your effort before it gets to the pedals)

STIFFNESS: Increases with density. Stiffer frames are often heavier.

WEIGHT: Lightweight (depending on the quality of alloy)

GOOD FOR:
➤ Touring and long-distance endurance riders
➤ Entry-level riders who want an inexpensive but comfortable bike

TITANIUM

Titanium (Ti) is another modern wonder material. It is extremely lightweight, strong, and durable. It also happens to be the most elastic of all materials, so while a Ti bike will be very strong, it easily flexes and returns to its original shape. This gives the bike a snappy feel that gives you a little boost.

Because of its durability, it's practically bombproof. However, if an impact is severe enough to cause damage, a Ti frame is expensive to repair.

COST: Expensive

DURABILITY:
➤ Doesn't rust
➤ Extremely durable
➤ Very difficult to repair

RIDE QUALITY:
➤ Springy, lively, responsive
➤ Gives feedback from the road
➤ Less responsive (the elasticity absorbs your effort before it gets to the pedals)

STIFFNESS: Lowest of all materials. Some manufacturers increase stiffness by shaping the tubing.

WEIGHT: Lightweight

BEST FOR:
➤ Riders who want a lightweight ride with a very responsive road feel and have a budget over $2,000

very low, it's likely the type of material is low quality, so all the other categories will suffer—especially durability.

DURABILITY is often the most important factor second to cost. We want a good deal, but we want it to last.

RIDE QUALITY is how the bike "feels" as reported by most riders. Frames can feel stiff, lively, dead, cushy, twitchy, and a whole lot more.

STIFFNESS refers to how much flexibility is in each material. Generally, stiff bikes lose less of the energy you transfer to the pedals (making you more efficient). Flexible bikes generally give you more cushion, but also suck away your pedaling power. This can greatly affect the ride quality.

WEIGHT is how much the average frame weighs. Please remember that you can have a light frame, but if you have heavy components, it will all balance out. If weight is a concern, always weigh the entire bike.

"GOOD FOR" is a description to give you a sense of what type of cyclist typically rides the material.

CHAPTER 8

Time to Shop

Before You Go

Hopefully by now you have a good idea of what you're looking for in a ride, frame material, and components. Armed with this info, you might be inclined to head for the nearest Craigslist posting or yard sale, but it is highly recommended to make your first road bike purchase from a local bike shop. Used bikes may seem like a great deal, but if the components are worn out or the fit is wrong, you didn't save a bundle—you just made a bad investment.

Now that you have things narrowed down, do a little online homework before you venture out. Hit your local bike shop's website. These days, brick-and-mortar bike shops have great sites that can let you know what brands they carry, and whether they specialize in road bikes, offer professional fitting services and classes, or offer test rides. The more customer service the shop offers upfront, the better your experience there is likely to be. Look at forums and reviews and see what other riders have said about the bikes you may want to try. Most importantly, do not be tempted to buy a bike from an online retailer. You'll likely end up with an unassembled bike (nope, they don't come put together) that may not fit. Bad idea.

When You Get There

Bike shop employees are trained to help you find the right size and make recommendations. A well-trained staff will help form a relationship for the long term. This

The "Best" Bike Brand

A COMMON QUESTION IS, "IS THAT A GOOD BRAND?"

The truth is, as long as you avoid department store bikes and go to a brick-and-mortar bicycle shop, the brands will be reliable. If you're unsure, ask about the warranty that comes with it. Good brands offer good warranties.

A common assumption by new cyclists is that if you pick the "right" brand, your bike will be perfect for you. "Hey, my brother-in-law has three bikes and they're all Treks. He says that's the best brand. That's what I want." Nope. Not necessarily.

Make your choice by your goals, needs, and budget. Different brands of bikes will all fit your wallet and your body. Bikes in a similar price range come with similar quality parts, but each brand will change your body position slightly. Sometimes the bike size that works for you will change from one brand to another. Sound a little bit like jeans or shoe shopping? Yep.

That is why test-riding multiple bikes is the key to finding your dream ride.

doesn't mean you should buy the first bike you ride—in fact, you'll want to test-ride a few.

Each shop tends to carry a few specific brands. To explore a variety of rides, make sure to visit more than one shop. When you walk in the door, you should be greeted and treated respectfully. There is no excuse for a shop that doesn't seem interested in taking your money, and lucky for you there are lots of bike shops out there.

Your salesperson should ask some of the same questions from the pop quiz to get started. If not, use the quiz answers as a guide to let them know what you're looking for. They'll likely make some suggestions based on what you tell them, then may ask you to sit on the bike while it's stabilized in a bike trainer to make sure it's close to the proper fit. Don't discount a bike on color or style. If it fits you well, give it a spin before discounting it completely.

You might find the two of you have a lot in common.

CHAPTER 9

The Importance of Test-Riding

TEST-RIDING IS THE MOST IMPORTANT PART OF THE BUYING experience. The only way to tell if a bike truly fits is by riding it. Before buying new shoes, you try them on. They may rub your heel, be too narrow, or not have enough support—or they may be just what you were looking for.

Think of your new bike as an exceptionally nice pair of shoes. The right fit is something a salesperson or your brother-in-law can't tell you. Your body and heart, however, will know when the fit is right.

You wouldn't wear a tuxedo to a first date. Come dressed for the ride. You don't need to be wearing Lycra, but don't show up in a business suit or a skirt with sandals and expect to have a good experience. Wear comfortable clothing

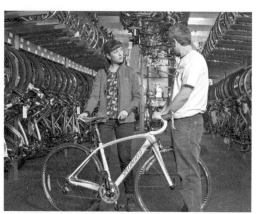

When you come to test-ride, wear comfortable clothing that you can move around in. If possible, bring bike shorts—that's the best way to know how the bike will feel when you're riding it.

you can easily move around in and get a little sweaty. It's a good idea to wear pants that taper at the ankle, or ask the shop for a strap to hold your pants safely out of the way of the chain.

Bring Your Wallet

If you want to head out of the shop to test-ride on the road, you'll need to hand over your driver's license and a valid credit card, no exceptions.

Get on an Even Playing Field

Before you hit the pavement, make sure you understand how the bike shifts and brakes. Different brands of components shift differently. A good shop will offer to show you how the shifters work in the store with the bike in a trainer. This way, you can concentrate on your ride rather than how to make the bike work.

You can't expect a (good) first date to last 15 minutes. Invest some time in your test-ride experience. It takes 20 to 30 minutes to have a conversation with the salesperson and for them to show you a few models, narrow them down to about the right fit, and then finally take them out for a ride. Plan on taking at least 15 to 30 minutes riding on the road for each bike. It takes close to that long to get a true feel for whether your body (arms, legs, back, etc.) is

getting sore anywhere. Yes, that means you could be in each shop for 2 to 3 hours, so this process may take more than a day.

Ask Questions and Make Adjustments

If this is your first road bike experience, you may think the salesperson has set the bike up for you. Then you ride and all your weight seems to be pressing into the saddle. Chances are the seat height is wrong. You may feel stretched out like Superman and can't reach the handlebars. Don't waste time on your full test ride if in the first few minutes it feels awful. Turn around and see if there is a simple adjustment the salesperson can make. That may work, or it may be the wrong fit. Don't discount what you feel just because you're a "newbie." If it feels wrong, it likely is wrong. If it's wrong, you won't want to ride it, so don't buy it.

A full bike fit breakdown is in the next section, so read ahead for more details on how a bike should fit.

She's an Uptown Girl . . .

Always test-ride a bike above and below your budget, even if you are certain you won't buy it. It will help you get a better sense of what you're paying for and how price affects quality.

CHAPTER 10

The Specifics of Women-Specific Design

FOLLOWING THE THEME OF BIKE FIT BEING SIMILAR TO clothing fit, it stands to reason that there should be offerings out there from the bicycle manufacturers that are made just for the ladies. But until about 15 years ago, women had one choice—a men's bike with which they could later swap out parts to make the best possible fit. A little like trying to steal your dad's shirt and rock it as "oversized chic."

As more women got on road bikes, research was done into how male and female bodies differ and how that might affect the bike they would want to ride. On average women have longer legs (usually in the thighbone), shorter torsos and arms, narrower shoulders, and smaller hands and feet. Of course, supporting the added upper body weight of breasts puts more strain on hands and wrists. Additionally, women have not only wider hips but also a deeper pelvis from front to back, which puts more pressure on their nether regions as their torso tilts forward to reach the handlebars.

So what to do? As the first bicycle manufacturers developed their bikes for women, they were known for "shrinking and pinking" men's bikes. They were using the same geometry and materials as traditional men's bikes—just in smaller sizes with a shorter stem, narrower and shallower handlebars with a shorter reach, and a slightly wider saddle. It was a good try, but solved only half of the actual fit differences—and not even the important ones.

As demand increased further and women became savvier shoppers, women-specific bicycles began to be designed with a tailored geometry that worked better for females. The top tube became "sloping," which angled it down toward the cranks and gave more room to stand over the frame. It was also shortened, which helped relax the reach to the handlebars. This was good news for short torsos, but made the front wheel so close to the pedals that you could hit it with your foot if you were pedaling while you turned (called toe overlap). Some manufacturers have compensated for this in

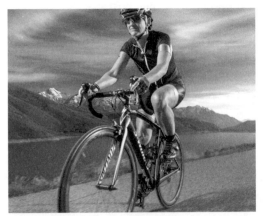
Women-specific bikes have come a long way in the past few years—and are sometimes a good fit for some men.

recent years, but some of the smallest frame sizes are still very tight.

At the same time, many manufacturers changed the angle of the seat tube to give longer-legged women more power than they ever had before. Stems that were already short became a little taller to help relieve pressure on the handlebars, and designers found ways to make the brake levers fit more diminutive hands. The smallest of bikes come with shorter crank arms. Saddles became not only wider, but also come with sections down the middle cut out to compensate for a deeper pelvis.

It's important to note that research also found that women have a much wider variety of body types and range of heights than men—which makes sizing females harder to generalize. All these women-specific designs were approximations for the "average" woman, so there are many female riders who will find themselves not fitting into this mold. As the ladies' lines developed, bikes for men started to be referred to as "unisex." Many women will find unisex bikes actually fit them better with a few tweaks. By the same token, occasionally there are men who—because of their height and proportions—find a woman-specific bike fits them better than a traditional unisex bike. Thankfully, after the first 10 years, the industry caught on that there was crossover, so they stopped making bikes for women with flowers, swirls, polka-dots, and pink handlebar tape. Now you can find both women-specific and unisex bikes in neutral colors.

CHAPTER 11

Upgrades and Add-Ons

NEW CYCLISTS OFTEN HAVE A CERTAIN EXPECTATION THAT since they plunked down thousands of dollars for a new bike, it will come equipped with everything they need. It's true for the most part—with the exception of pedals, your bike will likely come fully equipped.

But there are common (and less common) things you might want to invest a little more money in for your bike to have much better performance. They might have to do with the environment you're riding in or the type of riding you want to do. Unfortunately, bikes come stocked with the same parts no matter where you live or how you use your bike, so these tweaks to your ride can make a big difference.

One thing to be clear about is that these purchases will usually be upgrades as opposed to "trade-ins." Even as expensive as bicycles are, shops don't make much money selling them, so they usually can't afford to give you credit for the part that came on the bike that you hope to replace. Upgrades or add-ons mean you'll usually be paying full price for your new item. You can either sell the one that came with your bike, keep it as a backup, or donate it to your local bicycle nonprofit.

Pedals

It seems very obvious that a bike won't function well without pedals. That being said, most bikes over $1,200 don't come equipped with them because the industry got tired of throwing away pedals. Strange, huh? There are many, many brands and pedal systems on the market. Depending on the rider's style, physiology, and comfort on the road, he or she will usually have loyalty to a certain type or brand, so if a bike came stock with pedals he or she didn't like, they'd be tossed away. The solution? Bikes come as a blank slate to be filled in with your preference. So let's talk about your options.

The first type is what most of us have ridden our whole lives, *flat pedals*. They are named for the flat platform your foot easily finds to get the wheels turning. If it seems as if you wouldn't need more than that, think again. Your body can work most efficiently when you can control the pedal in a complete circle. With flat pedals, you are limited to only pushing down on the forward stroke of the pedal—using about one-fourth of the complete rotation your foot makes. Because of this, they are the least common on road bikes.

An improvement on the flat pedal came by way of *toe clips*. These are little cages on the front of the pedal that trap your toes and the ball of your foot to help you push down in the front of the pedal stroke and lift from the back,

giving you twice as much efficiency and power. You don't need special shoes, and the clips are fairly inexpensive (and removable). Their downfall is that in order to remove your foot, you have to pull back and out of the cage, which is sometimes hard to do—especially during an emergency stop when your body's weight is being propelled forward.

The final and most commonly used system today is called the *clipless pedal*. Its design is based on downhill-ski bindings, where your shoe has a cleat attached to it that locks into the pedal as you step down and releases when you twist your foot. Being "attached" to the bike may sound a little scary, but these are the most popular pedals for road bikes. They allow the rider to use the complete pedal stroke—gaining power around the entire rotation—making you faster and more efficient. Safety-wise, the pedal is quick and easy to release from the shoe with a flick of your foot, and in case of an accident your shoe will break free. These pedals are also smaller and therefore lighter than the flat option.

Clipless pedals are usually divided into two categories, mountain or road. Their names are deceiving though, because either can be used on a road bike and both regularly are. Each one was specifically developed for its type of riding, but later, riders found there was a lot of crossover. What they both have in common is an extremely stiff sole so that as much of your power as possible is transferred into the pedal—making you more efficient.

Mountain-style clipless pedals are often sold to new road cyclists when they begin riding because they are a great introduction to clipless pedals without sacrificing easy walking when off the bike. This style's benefits include being a little easier to clip in and out of, being able to clip in on both sides of the pedal, and having a cleat that sits deeper in the sole of your cycling shoe. This recessed cleat doesn't stick out at all, and you can pretty much walk in them the same as you would in a normal shoe. It was developed with the thought that mountain bikers sometimes have to hike on the trail to get around obstacles, or because their bike broke down in the middle of the woods. This pedal also works great for commuters and bike tourists who will be walking around in their shoes a lot when they are taking a break, or to get to their destination. The double-sided pedal also makes it much easier to clip in.

Overall, the contact points between pedal and shoe are small, giving your knee more side-to-side movement through the pedal stroke (called float), which can be a blessing for tricky knees. The downside is that it also decreases the amount of potential power and efficiency you could have. The very small area of contact can also cause "hot spots," which are places on the bottom of your foot that get painfully warm and uncomfortable after hours in the saddle.

Still, this system is much more efficient than flat pedals or those with toe cages.

The road-style clipless pedal uses a much larger cleat and pedal interface that utilizes more of the ball of your foot. Much like downhill-ski boots, the cleat on the shoe sticks out from the sole, forcing you to balance between your heel and the cleat when walking (and making your stride resemble an elf's). However, this design gives a huge power advantage over the mountain-style and is a good choice if you're putting on your shoes to walk out the door and get straight onto your bike, riding, then heading straight home, as you would for fitness or competitive riding.

Either way, if you decide to go clipless, be prepared for a steep but quick learning curve. A rite of passage when learning to ride clipless pedals is falling over when trying to get out of them. This almost always happens when coming to a dead stop while you're trying to put your foot down for balance while, say, waiting at a red light. You will tip over. You will be mostly unscathed, but your ego may be a little bruised if anyone notices. You are unlikely to be physically hurt or repeat this ever again.

To help avoid this scenario, ask your bike shop to install your cleats and adjust your pedals to the lowest spring tension setting before installing them. Practice clipping your bike shoe in and out of the pedals while the bike is stabilized in a trainer (which holds the bike upright and steady). This way you don't have to balance, brake, coast, or shift and you can get used to the feel of sitting on the bike and clipping in and out before you head out on the road. You'll be a pro in no time.

Saddles

This is the second-most common upgrade because fitting saddles is a little bit like fitting into jeans or shoes. Since everyone's anatomy and shape is a little different, size is only one part of the equation when you're shopping. For example, if you have a narrow foot, you might find that one brand of shoe fits better than another even though they are the same size. Then, of course, there's style to consider as well—though that tends not to make as big of a difference for most cyclists. Unlike jeans or shoes, the only way to tell if a saddle really fits is to spend at least an hour riding on it. Most quality bike shops will have a 30–day return policy on saddles because it will usually take that long to figure out if it fits or not.

We'll discuss saddles in greater detail in the next section, on bike fit, but keep in mind that when you first start riding, most every saddle will feel a little uncomfortable because your muscles aren't conditioned to the work and your bottom isn't conditioned to the pressure. If it still feels uncomfortable after the first month of long rides, or is causing distinct,

shooting pains not long into your ride, it's time to start looking around for a new saddle.

Tires and Tubes

One of the places that bicycle manufacturers will cut corners is by installing inexpensive, low-quality tires. Your first defense against getting punctures on the road is to upgrade to a higher performance or puncture-resistant tire. Since you're just getting started, we'll assume your main motivation is to avoid flats at all costs. Investing in some puncture-resistant tires can save you time and the cost of having to take your bike to the shop to fix your flat. But tires affect the quality of the ride, too. Inexpensive tires don't roll as smoothly and make going around corners and descending less safe because they don't grip the road as well.

In the case of living somewhere like the western United States, where desert thorns can be found on the road, you might want to invest in very puncture-resistant tires as well as tubes that are either thorn resistant or filled with a sealant. This sealant will fix small holes so you don't have to stop every time you hit a thorn or random blackberry. However, they do add significant weight to your ride, so consider how badly you need them before having the shop put them in.

If you're racing, you might look into spending a little extra on lighter, high-performance tires for race day. It might seem like a luxury to have tires you use for only a few days, but you can train on the lower quality tires that comes with the bike and then have a sweeter ride when it counts the most.

Wheels

Much like investing in a higher quality set of tires for race day, some people also want new wheels altogether. The wheels (and the tires) are among the heaviest parts of the bike because of the physics behind how they work. When spinning, it's as if the weight counts extra because you not only have to carry this weight forward down the road, but also around in a circle. This means more work for you if it's heavy.

The other reason some beginners may need to upgrade is if the wheels that come standard on the bike aren't tough enough. Unfortunately, most road bikes are built for riders under 225 pounds. If you weigh more than that or are planning on carrying enough weight that your total bike load will end up weighing that much, you might want to explore upgrading to a heavier wheel that will be less likely to be damaged under load.

PART IV

THE FIT

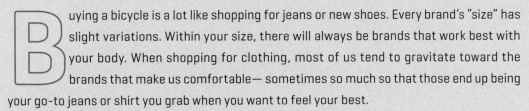

Buying a bicycle is a lot like shopping for jeans or new shoes. Every brand's "size" has slight variations. Within your size, there will always be brands that work best with your body. When shopping for clothing, most of us tend to gravitate toward the brands that make us comfortable— sometimes so much so that those end up being your go-to jeans or shirt you grab when you want to feel your best.

A properly fitting bike can—and should—have the same effect. After a while, it should disappear beneath you so you can concentrate on your ride, not your bicycle. Much like clothing, there are a lot of bikes that will fit you reasonably well right off the showroom floor. Fortunately, you can dial it in even more precisely by getting a professional bike fit. This is similar to having clothing you bought off the rack tailored to your exact specifications.

There are those riders who will have a hard time finding a good fit on the showroom floor, usually because their body is outside the spectrum of what most brands offer. These riders have the option of getting a bicycle custom made.

At the end of the day, there really is a perfect, fits-like-a-glove bike out there for each cyclist—often because you went the extra mile to make sure it was dialed in just for you.

CHAPTER 12

Why Good Fit Matters

SECOND TO YOUR ATHLETIC CONDITION, HOW THE BICYCLE
fits your body is the most important aspect of riding. You'll be spending a minimum of an hour in the saddle for many rides on a road bike—and the number one reason people don't meet their cycling goals is because they'll find this time increasingly painful. Some will end up abandoning the sport completely, while others may think they just need to "suck it up." Other than during the initial break-in period on your booty (usually 2 to 4 weeks depending on how often you're putting rubber to the road), there is no reason to put up with pain caused by the way the bike interacts with your body. Most of the time you're riding, your bike should disappear beneath you.

Bikes come in different sizes, which are intended as a guide. Brand to brand, the same size bikes change slightly in length and geometries, which is why test-riding to find the best brand for you is so important. Even a bike that's the right size may need to be adjusted to your body to properly fit for the most efficient and comfortable riding. Since all bodies—including their limitations and history of injuries—are different, it stands to reason that fit will vary quite a bit from rider to rider.

A bike that fits properly can mean the difference between a pain-free ride or possible long-term problems in your knees, neck, back, shoulders, elbows, wrists, hands, feet, or hips. That is a huge potential for injury when the main reasons you're riding to begin with are to feel healthier, enjoy the outdoors, and gain a little freedom from the doldrums of everyday life.

When thinking about fit, it's also important to consider what type of riding you hope to do. Bikes built for touring have the rider in a very upright position. There is a more aerodynamic position for recreational and fitness riders, and the position is lower still for racing. You may want to race, but your body's restrictions (such as a bad back or tight hamstrings) might call for a style that puts you in a more upright position. Be mentally flexible when it comes to where your body is most comfortable on a bike—it may not be what you envisioned, but it will keep you rolling longer.

Bike Fit 101

The two most important aspects of bike fit are seat height and reach. When you're shopping for a bike and sit on it for the first time, these are the two indicators that the size is cor-

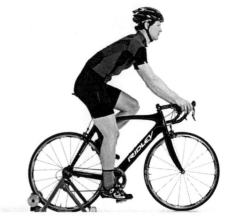

A properly fitting bike can make a world of difference in your comfort and efficiency.

rect. Above is a rough idea of how a bike should properly fit.

The seat should be high enough that you have a very slight bend in your knee when your foot is at the very bottom of the pedal stroke. This gives you the most power with the least chance of injury.

Your reach should be so that your arms and torso make a 45-degree angle over the bike. Too long and it will be hard to reach the handlebars; too short and your knees will be too close to your arms and your back will arch.

CHAPTER 13

Taking It to the Tailor: Professional Bike Fit and Fitters

Having Your Bicycle Tailor-Fit

While bike shopping, you're trying to find the closest size that will work for you. When you buy your new bike, the salesperson may put your bike in the trainer and adjust the seat height. Sometimes he'll even swap out a stem. Then he'll pat you on the back, tell you they "fit" you, and send you off on your merry way.

Don't be misled. This is not a professional bike fit.

A professional fit is something you'll schedule with your bike shop and takes from an hour and a half to more than 2 hours to complete. The fitter will take time to discuss your style of riding and goals for the future. Next, he may take you through a series of tests to test your flexibility and core strength. Finally, he will seat you on your bike or a special fitting cycle to put together all the information he has gathered, then make adjustments to your bike and swap out parts you may need.

If you spent more than $1,000 on an off-the-rack suit, you'd likely get it professionally tailored. Your bike, like the suit, is off the show-room floor. In both cases, you want your new purchase to move smoothly, without chafing, pain, or any awkwardness. When road riding, you'll be spending many hours in a position that's new to you and your body, so it's important that the bike fits correctly.

That being said, you can wear any clothes or ride any bike and put up with bad fit. But the difference between clothes and your bike is that clothes that don't fit will wear out in funny places and perhaps look unattractive, which while sad, isn't really hurting anything. If your bicycle doesn't fit well, you'll be the one wearing out—from pain, numbness, and fatigue.

Each of us comes with our own set of injuries, limitations, and special sizing quandaries. Let's say riders A and B have just bought the exact same bike and are within a half-inch of each other in height. Rider A is 24 years old, is looking to race bikes, and has really huge feet. Rider B is 60, has had multiple back surgeries, has a very broad upper torso, and bought his bike to ride in organized recreational rides. Same bike—but totally different fit needs.

An aggressive posture that slopes down from the saddle to the handlebars may suit rider A well. He'll also need his seat and cleats positioned forward or backward to compensate for his large shoe size. Rider B may need to be more upright to help alleviate back pain (from both the surgery and the lack of flexibility that usually comes with age) and give him more room to chat with his riding buddies. His handlebars may get swapped out for something a little wider to ward off shoulder pain. But these are only guesses, because until a professional fitter works with them, there's no telling how much more powerfully, efficiently, and comfortably these guys could be riding.

It's good to put some miles on your bike before you make the appointment. Riding at least 150 to 200 miles will let you know where your body isn't feeling its best, help you find out if the saddle is working for your butt, and gain some muscle memory to use for comparison after your fit.

Professional Bike Fitters

Bike shops are great places to find both fitters and the professional bicycle mechanics who will check the work for safety after fitters install parts.

The shop will also have a stock of stems, saddles, and other replacement parts you may need and should be a part of any professional fitting service. It's extremely important because it's the only way to correct many common problems (saddle fit, leg positioning, reach to the handlebars).

Sometimes a physical therapist or chiropractor will offer a professional bike-fitting service from their medical office, but they may not be able to supply parts. Although it may seem like a good idea to go to a medical professional, it can be a waste of time and money if they don't have access to the parts you'll need and, more importantly, don't have the mechanical know-how to safely swap out the old components for new ones. Occasionally a bike shop or other cycling facility will have a partnership with a medical professional, giving you access to the best of both worlds.

Look for a bicycle shop that requires its bicycle fitters to have a minimum of 40-plus hours of training before they start to work with customers. Many fitters have a background in physical therapy, massage, or racing, all of which can give them an edge.

Finally, if you've decided you want to race, look for a fitter who has experience working with racers or has raced. Conversely, if you're mainly planning on using your bicycle for touring, this same fitter may not be your best choice. If you live somewhere with a large selection of bicycle stores, shop around online for prices and recommendations and inquire with the bike shop about their fitters' experience before you make an appointment.

CHAPTER 14

The Fit Experience: What to Expect

FIRST OF ALL, BE FOREWARNED: BIKE FIT CAN BE A PRETTY intimate experience. Your fitter will be interacting with your body, sometimes even moving you around or asking you to lie on the floor for a flexibility test. You may have to relive past physical traumas when you share your injury history. That broken wrist from when you fell off your skateboard when you were 16 can make a difference when it comes to hours of pressure when your hands rest on the handlebars.

Come prepared. Make a mental list of all your previous injuries—even the ones that may have happened years ago—and strengths. Wear what you will be riding in, as it will affect both your seat height and foot position. Be prepared to challenge what you might have thought a proper fit meant and focus on your own body. The fitter can see how your body interacts with the bicycle, but in the end it's up to your personal comfort level. Keep in mind, the goal is to improve how you feel on the bike and how strong and efficient you are.

When you arrive, the fitter will have you change into your riding gear (if you're not already wearing it). He may test your flexibility and take measurements of different parts of your body.

Next, he'll secure your bike in a trainer or ask you to sit on one of the special bike-fitting tools (which looks like a very funny stationary bike) and have you pedal. He'll be examining your pedal stroke, how you sit on your saddle, your hip position, the angle of your torso and arms, and how your shoulders, arms, and wrists look resting on the bars. Based on what you've explained about your body and its strengths and limitations, he may make changes in some of the following areas. This will take time, as your fit on the bike is dynamic, so changing one area will often affect others that will have to be adjusted in turn. For example, moving the seat forward to make an adjustment for your knee may create a need for your handlebars to be moved forward as well and the cleat to be adjusted differently on your shoe.

Reach to your handlebars is how far your hands have to go to rest on the bars. If it's too short or long, you'll want to put the weight of your hands on the wrong part of the bar, making it hard to shift or brake the bike. This can be fixed by installing a different length and/or angle of stem, or depth and/or width of handlebar.

Hand position has two major factors. One is how wide your handlebars are. Depending on how broad your shoulders and back are, it can be adjusted with a wider or narrower bar. The other is how close the brake lever is to reach for the rider. Some components have a small screw that allows the lever to come in closer for small hands. Others use a tiny shim to shorten the brake lever reach.

Saddle position has many factors, all of which can influence other parts of the fit. The most obvious and common change will be seatpost height. Even something as little as a centimeter change can mean the difference between shooting knee pain and a comfy ride. It's also common to move the seat forward or backward to help situate your hips, knees, and feet into a proper alignment. Seat width and length vary greatly between different saddle manufacturers. The bones in your pelvis can't be supported if the seat is too narrow or wide. We'll discuss in-depth how to buy a saddle on the next page.

Finally, *leg and cleat position* helps you get the most power out of pedaling.

If you've decided to use clipless pedals, the cleat attachment points on the bottom of the shoe are adjustable. When you buy the shoes and pedals, the bike shop will install them in a neutral position. However, that doesn't mean it's anywhere close to being the right angle or placement for your foot since everyone's bodies (even from one side to another) differ so much.

All these factors have tons of tiny adjustments to be made within them. This is why it's

Frequently Replaced or Additional Parts

➤ **Stem:** The stem affects your reach. It is probably the most common part to be swapped out since many riders have longer or shorter torsos or arms compared to the average that the bike manufactures built the bike around. ($20–$250, with an average being around $40)

➤ **Handlebars:** The width and depth of the handlebars also affects your reach. ($40–$300)

➤ **Shims:** These are tiny wedges that sit inside your shifters and help bring the brake lever closer to the handlebar for smaller hands. ($5–$10)

➤ **Seatpost:** Some posts have seat attachment points that will help bring the saddle forward or back. ($20–$200)

➤ **Saddles (Seats):** The other most commonly changed part of the bike. They are very individual to the rider. After an hour in the saddle, your bottom will tell you if the fit is right. ($40–$400)

➤ **Cables:** If a stem or handlebar swap makes the reach significantly farther away, all your cables may need to be replaced with longer ones. ($20–$60— labor to change them is sometimes not included)

➤ **Bar Tape:** Some bodies need more padding in the handlebar tape to help absorb shock. It's common to either upgrade to a softer, thicker tape or put a thin layer of vibration-absorbing material underneath your bar tape to increase the cushioning.

especially important to find an experienced, professional bicycle fitter. This is also why the cost of bike fitting tends to be $150 to $250. This covers not only the initial fit, but also any follow-up you might need. However, it does not include any of the parts you'll be swapping out, which are considered "upgrades" and can add quite a bit of cost to your fitting.

If all goes well, you may not return for another visit. However, since most of the bike fit is done in a stationary setting (like a bike trainer), it's hard to know if everything is dialed in until you go out and try the bike on the road with your new positioning. Any quality bike fitter should have a guarantee that you'll be satisfied with your fit or he will keep working with you until it's right. It's not unusual to go back after your initial fit to make small tweaks.

What's in a Seat?

Bicycle saddles (or seats) may seem deceptively simple, but because so much is literally riding on it, it's one of the most important and personal items on your bike. Your booty and your groin are at stake, so finding the right fit is key.

Let's take shoes for example. You wouldn't walk around in the wrong size shoes—your feet would soon be covered in blisters. Nor would you put on dress shoes to go for a jog. Serious runners use footwear that can help support their stride and help their muscles work most

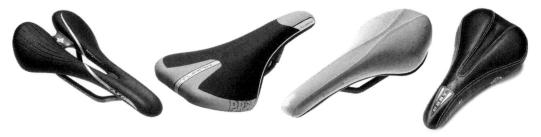

Bike saddles can vary widely in shape and size (just like us).

efficiently, and they make sure the size is right. The same is true for the seat on your bike. Unfortunately, there are almost as many types and styles of saddles on the market as there are shoes—and not all of them are designed to be used for the longer miles that most road cyclists will be putting in. Trickier still, although there are ways to measure the length, width, and arch of your foot, that's not the case with a bike seat—it's mostly left to trial and error.

The shape of a road saddle may seem a little odd but is actually quite brilliant. Most saddles have a triangular shape with two long rails running beneath it that connect to your seatpost. Since your goal is to spin your legs at 90 to 100 rotations per minute, this narrow design leaves your muscles room to move freely. The slightly wider rear of the saddle is suspended over the rails, creating a hammock-like support system for your pelvis that has some give in it to help absorb the bumps in the road while allowing air to flow beneath your seat. The forward bending of your torso in a road bike position allows you to spread your body weight between your hands and feet as well, so the saddles on road bikes tend to be longer and more narrow than other more upright styles of bikes because they aren't taking as much of your weight and what they are supporting is contacting on a slightly different angle.

If you sat down on a hard bench or stair, you'd likely start to feel sore on the two bumps that protrude from your bottom, commonly referred to as your "sit bones." On a bicycle seat, these are the points that make the most contact with your bike saddle. When the saddle properly fits you, those points will bear most of the weight so that the delicate soft tissues between them don't get compressed—which is one of the leading causes of discomfort.

Speaking of which, the nose (or front end) of the saddle is there to help with balance and control of the bike. It does its job well, but it is also the place where most cyclists get pain, numbness, or irritation because it's right where all the soft tissue compresses. To alleviate this problem, many saddles are designed with a long depressed section in the middle to create more room. Others go so far as to make a long oval hole or a channel cutout so that there's little to interfere with your soft bits.

As far as thickness goes, new riders will often gravitate to a more padded saddle, thinking it will prevent soreness. Not so. Because your thighs need room for movement, a lot of padding can cause chafing and irritation. If you think back to our example of sitting on a hard stair or bench, imagine putting a piece of nice, squishy foam beneath you. Sounds nice, but because you likely weigh 120-plus pounds, after a few minutes your bones have sunk back to the cement and the padding will have worked itself *between* your sit bones, compressing all your vulnerable soft tissue—exactly what you want to avoid.

There are saddles specifically designed for both men and women, but because of the wide range of variation in the human anatomy, there is often crossover. In general, men's pelvises are shallower from front to back (which gives them more room to rotate their pelvis forward and tilt toward the handlebars) and the space between their sit bones is smaller. Front to back, women's pelvises are deeper and more bowl shaped and their sit bones are spread farther apart. Because of this, men's saddles are usually designed to be more narrow and longer than women's.

Unfortunately, there's no magic formula for seat fitting—but this is also where an experienced bicycle fitter can earn every penny. By looking at your pedal stroke and hearing you describe how you're feeling and where your

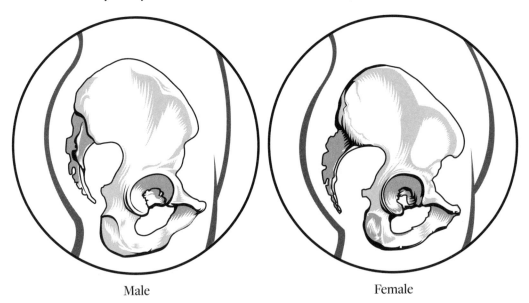

Male   Female

The differences between a man's and a woman's pelvis can affect bike fit and saddle selection. Women's pelvises are often wider (which affects seat width) and deeper (allowing less room for the torso to bend forward to reach the handlebars).

pain is, he can make educated recommendations. Professional bicycle fitters are also usually the most well versed in what saddles are available on the market—and which work the best—because they are constantly getting feedback on saddle fit.

Finally, a little reality check. If this is your first time riding a bike in a long while, your booty is going to be sore. *No* saddle will fix this, but a saddle that fits will become so comfortable that it will eventually feel like it disappears beneath you. Your muscles surrounding and beneath your sit bones will need to build up strength and resistance. It will probably be quite a few rides before your bum is in compliance with what you're asking of it. Start with short rides—no more than 5 to 15 miles. Over a few weeks' or months' time, work up to riding an hour. Try to ride at least twice a week or each ride will be like starting from scratch. Be patient, and shortly enough saddle soreness will usually dissipate.

If after a good amount of riding the discomfort hasn't disappeared (or seems to be getting worse the longer you're in the saddle), you'll need to start looking for a new seat. Any reputable shop should have a 30-day return policy on its saddles so you have time to get a few rides of at least an hour in and decide if it's working for you. If it's not right, bring it back and try another. It might take a few attempts, but your derrière will thank you for it. In the end you won't really know if a saddle is right for you until you spend time riding it.

CHAPTER 15

Custom Bikes: Having It Your Way

CUSTOM BICYCLES HAVE BEEN AROUND SINCE THE BEGINNING of the industry, when one builder's hands welded each bike for one particular customer. Custom bikes never really went away completely, and for many decades the techniques were kept alive by a few artisans in the United States and Europe. However, in the past 10 years there's been a huge resurgence of custom builders, especially in the United States. Now you can easily find at least a few and sometimes as many as 10 to 20 to choose from in every state.

What makes custom bikes special—and expensive—is that the tubes are hand cut and welded to your specifications, usually by one builder. Want a rack built in for touring? The fastest road bike around? Special sizing? An experience that's catered to your every need? A custom bicycle is the epitome of making your riding dreams come true.

As we've already covered, some bodies don't fall so neatly into a "women-specific" or "unisex" box. Both these designs are based on the average found in the middle of a bell curve. But what to do if you if you're an outlier?

A professional fit can help, but sometimes even after replacing all the components you possibly can, you'll still be left with a fit that's less desirable. Square pegs will never fit into round holes, which is one reason custom bicycles came back into fashion.

The other reason is that some riders want to commandeer a bike that isn't just professionally fit. They want the full-meal deal—the ultimate experience of having a bike designed around their body type, riding style, and fit, and then have the icing on the cake of being able to choose their own color.

Welcome to the world of custom bicycles.

Beginner riders will find this experience either mind-bendingly overwhelming or perfectly suited to their tastes. The upside of having a custom bike is that you get to choose every component and dream up every detail. The downside is you have the responsibility of making those choices. If you're not confident in choosing what is best for you when it comes to your ride, you might be quickly overwhelmed with deciding which tires, shifters, brakes,

cranks, pedals, and so on suit you best. You can expect some guidance from the builder in these matters, but don't blame the messenger if you end up not liking what he picked out for you.

As far as fit goes, any quality custom builder should expect that you'll be sized with a professional bike fit before he starts the build. He may farm this out to another professional fitter or offer to do the fit himself. A custom builder should never base a bike build on a bike you're currently riding—unless you want to end up with some of the same problems you may already be experiencing. The only way to be close to the correct fit is to have your body sized before the tubes are cut and welded.

Custom bikes are often something that come after a rider has had experience with massproduced bicycles and is now more dialed in to his or her own needs and preferences. However, if your body is very tall or extremely small, you're likely already familiar with having to go the extra mile to find clothing or shoes that work. Custom bicycles are just an extension of this concept, and although they may cost you a bit more, they'll be worth every penny in performance on the road and prevention of pain and injury.

PART V

GEARING UP FOR SUCCESS

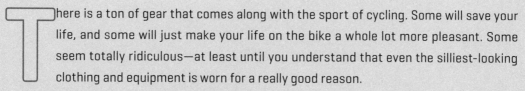

There is a ton of gear that comes along with the sport of cycling. Some will save your life, and some will just make your life on the bike a whole lot more pleasant. Some seem totally ridiculous—at least until you understand that even the silliest-looking clothing and equipment is worn for a really good reason.

At first glance, your average road cyclist may look—and sometimes walk—a little funny. That's because the attire is designed for high performance and optimal safety.

CHAPTER 16

Dress for the Occasion: The Basics

THINK YOU DON'T NEED SPECIAL CLOTHING TO RIDE? YOU'RE (mostly) right. With the exception of always including a helmet, you really can ride in anything. However, technical bicycle clothing helps keep you safe, comfortable, and faster on the road. Bike clothing designers have spent many years tweaking and refining these products, and they've come a long way. Yes, they look a little silly, and you may be a bit intimidated to embrace the Lycra—especially since most of us associate it with 1980s aerobics classes and it doesn't leave much to the imagination. But take a look and hear us out on why you should consider making the leap into the wonderful world of spandex.

Materials

Most bicycle clothing is made from materials that are made to dry quickly and wick perspiration away from your skin. This is extremely important because as you're riding, any moisture in your clothing can cause chafing and irritation—not to mention that riding around in damp clothing makes you clammy and leaves you smelling not so fresh.

The two most common fabrics are high-tech poly mixes and merino wool. Both materials wick sweat and are quick drying, but the high-tech polyester mixes are more common and affordable.

Merino wool is not your granddad's sweater material. It's nature's miracle fiber that is highly durable, wicks, insulates (keeping you cool in the summer and warm in the winter, depending on the thickness), dries quickly, and has antimicrobial properties that keep your clothes from building up with "gym stink." Unfortunately there are only so many merino sheep (found mainly in New Zealand) and it costs quite a bit more to farm than to spin materials out of polyester, so their resulting material is much more expensive.

Jersey

This is your bike shirt. It comes in short-sleeved, long-sleeved (for the winter), or ladies' sleeveless variations (for the summer). From the front, it looks like a regular tight shirt, but it is actually a well-thought-out piece of clothing that is defined by a few key design components.

Jerseys are intended to be worn snugly to

help keep you aerodynamic. How sleek you are may not seem like a big deal at first, but it makes a huge difference in how much effort you'll need to put out while riding. So while you may be tempted to wear something a little less form-fitting, consider that you'll be making your ride a little tougher by doing so.

The jersey is cut longer in back and shorter in front to accommodate your bent-over riding position. This adds to the awkward look when you're just walking around, but covers your lower back and keeps material from binding up or cinching in the front when you're on the bike. The front also has a three-quarter to full-

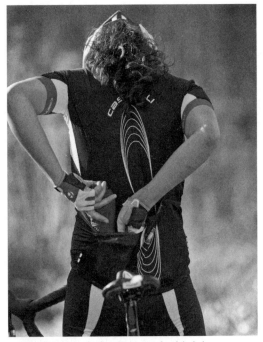

Jersey pockets tucked away on your back help keep you aerodynamic and prepared for the ride.

length zipper to give you extra ventilation when needed.

Another technical aspect of the jersey is the back pockets. You'll want one with at least three. There are jerseys with fewer, but most riders find that they want as much space as possible to carry all the things they may find themselves needing, including food, water, on-the-road repair items, sunscreen, jackets, and more. This clever placement not only keeps your stuff where you can easily reach it while you're riding without it falling out, but also keeps it tucked out of the way of the wind. Since this is really the only viable place for pockets on the bike, the pockets are truly essential.

For strict cycle-tourists or commuters who have other means of carrying the things you need (like saddle bags or a backpack), a true cycling jersey may not be necessary, though you'll still want to wear some kind of material that wicks perspiration. There are cycling shirts that look a little more like everyday wear (no back jersey pockets) but that are made of good materials and are cut slightly better for cycling.

Bike Shorts and Chamois Time

Bike shorts are made of the "slimming" Lycra that most people envision when they think of cyclists. Though commonly referred to as shorts, they also come in three-quarter-length and full-length versions (usually referred to as tights) for cooler-weather riding.

The shorts are usually made of multiple panels of material to help create the most smooth, snug, and comfortable fit. When you're shopping, the higher the panel count, the more expensive and well fitting the shorts usually are.

You'll also have a choice of whether to get bibs or regular shorts. Regular shorts have a waistband that can be a source of discomfort because you'll be bent over the whole time you're on the bike. The bibs make you look like a high school wrestler (at least when your jersey is off) but eliminate the rolling and bind-

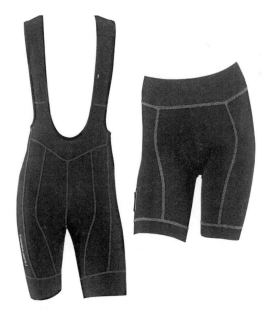

Shorts or bibs are both good options on the bike.

Mentioning the Unmentionables

A WORD ABOUT UNDERWEAR: AS FAR AS bottoms go, you won't wear any because your shorts and chamois will do the job for you. If you try to wear them underneath your chamois, not only will you have horrid panty or brief lines, you're going to be in for a very rough ride. In fact, the whole point of how bicycle shorts are designed is to prevent the unseemly sores that can be caused by underwear. So leave them behind.

As for the ladies, your basic fitness sports bras are highly recommended. As with any sports activity, your chest needs the wicking properties they provide as well as protection from road vibration and bumps along the way, so keeping them firmly braced against your body is best.

ing of the waistband through the use of over-the-shoulder straps. This can make bathroom breaks a little tricky because of the need to remove your top to get your bibs off (men have more options for getting around this). However, most riders find that this minor inconvenience is well worth the extra comfort in the long haul. One fashion note—bib straps are intended to be worn under your jersey, not over it.

Sewn inside is the chamois (commonly pronounced "shammy"), a big padded liner that protects your behind from soreness and chafing. The word originates from the goatlike animal whose skin was the fabric for the first liners ever used—and back in the day these worked surprisingly well for decreasing friction on riders' bottoms. Lucky for us, the modern chamois is made from some combination of foam and gel and is covered with a microfiber cloth that wicks away sweat. Beware of getting the thickest chamois thinking it will offer the most protection. If the padding is too thick, it can actually cause numbness and lose its beneficial quick-drying properties.

For commuters who may not be riding for hours at a time and sometimes ride in their work clothes, there are thin liners to be worn under your "regular" clothes that have a thin chamois. This works a bit like the regular bike shorts but without the bulk—and you can wear them all day long if you like.

Shoes and Socks

Your shoes will mostly depend on what type of pedals you've chosen to ride. If you've decided to ride flat pedals, any fitness or gym shoe will work fine, though the stiffer the sole, the more power that can be transferred from your body to the pedal, so some shoe companies offer a shoe that works fairly well.

If instead you've decided to go with a clipless pedal system, your choice of shoes will be based on whether you decided on the road or mountain type of pedal. The mountain cleat attaches with two bolts, the road cleat with three, so generally you'll need road shoes for road-specific pedals, and mountain shoes for mountain-specific pedals. (See more detailed descriptions of your pedal choices in Chapter 11.) With either kind the fit should be somewhat snug around your foot—not too tight, but as narrow as your foot will allow. This helps transfer power and keep you aerodynamic.

Cycling-specific socks are made of special wicking fibers and are designed to give support in the arch, to provide padding where you need it, and not to bunch up or rub. Of course, there are varying lengths to choose from, but the height of the cuff has little to do with functionality and everything to do with fashion. From preventing tan lines to the current trend in cycling sock fashion, your choice of sock length is highly personal.

Helmets

Technically, helmets make everyone look slightly insect-like. It's true. However, they're the most important and valuable item you'll put on to ride a bike. Riders shouldn't saddle up without reaching for their helmets first. There is never a reason to go for a ride—even a quick jaunt to the coffee shop or park—without a helmet on. Of all the parts of your body that can break, your brain is the most valuable and least repairable.

Yes, the chances are slim that you'll fall. Unfortunately, if you do it's never expected. Because of the riding position, it's difficult, if not impossible, to protect your head in case of an accident without a helmet. Even when you're not moving quickly (many falls are surprisingly slow or even come from losing your balance at a dead stop), it's all too easy to bump your head on the pavement or curb if you go down.

All helmets sold in bike shops meet the same levels of safety certification standards whether they cost $40 or $300. The main difference is that the more expensive helmets are much lighter and have better ventilation and more high-tech bells and whistles for adjustment without compromising on safety. So if you're resistant to wearing a helmet because you love the feeling of the wind in your hair, invest in a higher-end helmet so you can enjoy the wind and keep your best asset safe.

Replace your helmet:

➤ If you fall
➤ If you drop it regularly
➤ If the outer shell is compromised with dents or cracks
➤ Every 2 to 3 years. UV rays from the sun and age deteriorate the integrity of the helmet. Even if you kept it in a

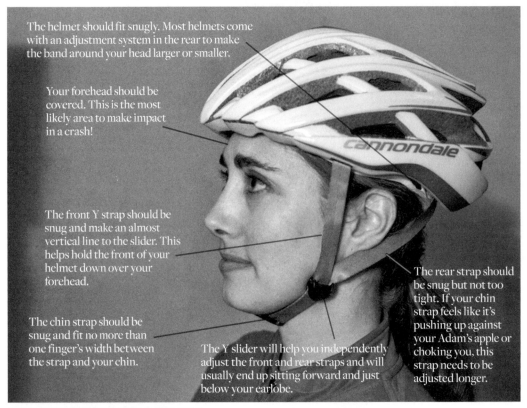

The helmet should fit snugly. Most helmets come with an adjustment system in the rear to make the band around your head larger or smaller.

Your forehead should be covered. This is the most likely area to make impact in a crash!

The front Y strap should be snug and make an almost vertical line to the slider. This helps hold the front of your helmet down over your forehead.

The chin strap should be snug and fit no more than one finger's width between the strap and your chin.

The Y slider will help you independently adjust the front and rear straps and will usually end up sitting forward and just below your earlobe.

The rear strap should be snug but not too tight. If your chin strap feels like it's pushing up against your Adam's apple or choking you, this strap needs to be adjusted longer.

HOW TO PROPERLY FIT A HELMET
If your helmet doesn't fit right, it's not safe. Make sure you not only wear it, but also have it adjusted properly.

closet, replace helmets that are older than 3 years.

A properly fitting helmet should feel snug like a baseball cap. Head sizes and shapes vary, so if it feels loose or tight in the proper size, try a different brand.

1. Not too far forward
2. Not too far back
3. Tighten back clamp
4. Adjust sliders
5. Adjust buckle

CHAPTER 17

Protect Your Assets: Staying Comfortable

NOW THAT WE HAVE COVERED THE BASICS OF CYCLING GEAR, it's time to up the ante and discuss another realm of equipment. We'll get into the extra stuff you might need to keep you protected from the elements, road conditions, and even a spill or a swarm of insects.

Cold is a terrible force and heat can be just as bad. Cyclists need barriers from the outside and layers from the inside to help keep temperatures manageable, so the industry has designed products you can add or take away while riding as weather conditions change. Remember those jersey pockets we talked so much about? One of their main functions is to stow away the various clothing and accessories you may need as a spring day turns from beautiful to nasty and back again, so you can be prepared no matter what the world throws at you.

Most of the following items are not things every cyclist buys off the bat, but they may be acquired over time as the needs arise. If you know you're only able to ride cold early mornings, a windbreaker might be one of your first purchases. A commuter might need lights, or a cycle-tourist may want chamois cream for those long days in the saddle. Which of these items you want to invest in will depend on your riding style, your budget, and your priorities.

Layering: Building from the Inside Out

Whether the conditions are hot or chilly, or even if it's the perfect summer day, there are a few things you can count on to keep you both warm, cool, and abrasion-free.

Base Layers

Cyclists cannot underestimate the power of the base layer. How can a fancy undershirt make that big of a difference? Let's start with the cold. Two thin layers are lighter and better insulated than a thicker one because the space between them traps some of the warmth your body creates. It's hard to believe, but a base layer will do more to keep your extremities warm than a thick pair of gloves or socks. Adding protection to your extremities will help, of course. But keeping your torso warm keeps the majority of the blood in your body warmer, which in turn keeps your extremities from getting too cold in the first place.

This is where the magic is—around the core, where most of all your temperature is regulated. Starting from your heart, blood expands out to your extremities. Think of it like the furnace or AC in your house. There's the main unit (your heart, lungs, and innards), vents that push cold or warm air out (your arteries), and vents that reclaim the old air to be cycled again (your veins). So even if you have a room that's built off a wing of the house (like your hands or feet), it comes down to regulating the central system for good temperature control throughout your proverbial house.

"But I'm sweating!" some say. "I must be warm enough!" Sweat worked up on a climb doesn't always mean your core temp is warm enough to keep you toasty on the downhill. A fine-tuned body should sweat when your heart rate rises. This doesn't mean you can stay warm enough to keep your extremities from turning to icicles, so protect that precious resource with some insulation. The best material for the winter base layer is merino wool because of its fabulous wicking and insulating properties.

There are also "cooling" base layers for hot days. Seems a little counterintuitive, but the explanation is based on the science surrounding your body's natural mechanism. Sweat's main job is to cool your body by using your own core heat to help evaporate water on your skin. The more you sweat, the more warmth your body releases to evaporate the moisture away. So in normal or humid climates, cooling base layers can be helpful because they keep your core temp from overheating by moving some of the water off your skin for you. These base layers are usually made from synthetics or bamboo.

Take note: In drier climates you want to avoid the cooling base layer. It can remove the sweat from your skin too quickly before it has a chance to draw any heat out, leaving your core temperature too high.

Chamois Cream

Sounds a little curious, huh? Your chamois is made to wick sweat, but on hot days it can only wick so much. Combine that with the fact that you'll be pedaling circles around 90 times a minute (which is 45 times for each leg), and in an hour you've brushed each leg about 2,700 times against the saddle. That's quite a bit, so you can see how chafing can be a problem—especially if you're in the saddle for longer.

This is where chamois cream comes in. It is a thick cream that provides a protective layer between the friction points where the edges of the saddle hit your bum. After a few rides, this spot will easily identify itself. If you're experiencing rawness—something akin to a burn—on your bottom after rides, chamois cream will help prevent it and can even be used off the saddle to help it heal. The cream is also a preventative against the horrors of saddle sores. These are little spots of irritation that turn into infected hair follicles caused by the bacteria in your sweat. Unlike the aforementioned abrasion, these can be a lot more painful and take

days or weeks to heal. No fun at all, and difficult if not impossible to ride a bike comfortably while you have one.

There are numerous chamois creams out there that your bicycle shop should carry. There are also non-cycling products that work for some, but they are either too greasy or absorb too quickly. After comparative testing, many people usually find a type and brand that they prefer. Caution—some brands come with mentholated "cooling" or "tingly" versions (sometimes referred to as "Euro style"). If you have sensitive skin, read the labels carefully.

Barriers: Protecting from the Outside In

Whether you're rolling out in the morning cold or the forecast says to expect the unexpected, these are the things you can wear to keep the elements from destroying your ride—or your body afterward.

Jackets and Vests

Jackets and vests seem like simple items, but like jerseys, cycling jackets are unique. They are also cut longer in the back than they are in front and are usually designed to either protect from wind, the cold, rain, or all three, each one being progressively thicker and less breathable than the one before.

Windbreakers are ultrathin, lightweight, and

usually designed to easily pack into one of your jersey pockets so you can wear it when you need it, then stow it away. To make them as packable as possible, they usually come without pockets. Imagine a jacket that can fold down to the size of a soda can and you're in the ballpark. That being said, their ability to stop the wind from creeping down to your base layer and cooling your skin is second to none. Even on a 70-degree day, a long, shady descent at 30 miles per hour can be bone-chilling, so pull it out of your pocket before the descent and then tuck it away when you're back on flat ground. Of course, on a colder day, a wind jacket (with proper layering beneath) is all you might need for the whole ride. As far as breathability, these usually don't leave much room for your body to breathe, so the jacket can make you overheat quickly and is best removed if you don't really need it. If you're riding when it's below 75 degrees and your ride has a long descent, it's a must have.

A vest is a variation on this. It has all the same qualities as the jacket, but without sleeves. Similar to a base layer, it works by keeping your core at its warmest, but differs in that it leaves your arms exposed so they stay drier. If you're a person who tends to run warm or perspires a lot, this might be a better choice than a full windbreaker for most of your rides. For anyone on a spring day when the warm hasn't quite set in, it can be a perfect piece of your wardrobe.

Fend Off the Elements

ALTHOUGH MOST ROAD BIKES AREN'T built to accommodate fenders, it doesn't mean you have to ride around with a droopy, soggy chamois or that you have to spray the rider behind you with a face full of grit. If you're riding in bad weather, these can be your best defense against being miserable.

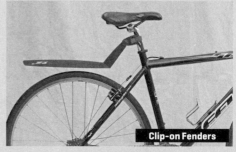
Clip-on Fenders

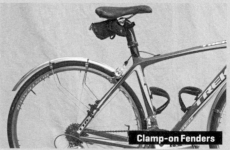
Clamp-on Fenders

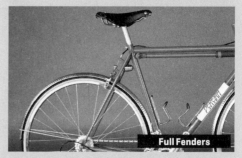
Full Fenders

The type of fender you choose will mostly depend on what kind of road bike you're riding.

CLIP-ON FENDERS

STRAP AROUND THE SEATPOST, ARC behind the rear wheel, and protect your backside. Some come with a front option, but many don't.

Pros:
- Easy installation for even the least mechanically inclined
- Easily removed
- Transferable from one bike to another
- Inexpensive

Cons:
- Many don't come with a front fender option.
- Have the least amount of coverage
- Won't fit on some seatposts and will scratch carbon fiber

CLAMP-ON FENDERS

COVER MORE OF THE CIRCUMFERENCE of your front and rear wheels, leaving you slightly more protected from the wet and grime.

Pros:
- Fairly easy to install or remove (most strap on to your bike frame with a heavy-duty rubber-band enclosure)
- Better coverage on front and rear
- Lightweight

Cons:
- Finicky and shift easily, needing regular micro-adjustments to not rub against your wheel
- Can leave scratches on your lovely paint job if you don't use protective tape where it attaches to the frame

FULL FENDERS

THE ULTIMATE OPTION FOR PROTECTING yourself from a soggy bum and street grit in your eye. They bolt into your bike, making them sturdy and semipermanent. Available in both plastic (more economical) or metal (classier, but heavier and more expensive).

Pros:
- The best coverage of any option, will keep you the most clean and dry
- Once properly installed, don't need much adjusting
- Are not easily removed, so theft is not a problem

Cons:
- Depending on your bike, they can be extremely fussy and time consuming to install, so many cyclists find it's worth the money to have a professional mechanic handle the job.
- More expensive than other options
- Most modern road bikes do not have enough room to fit full fenders without having to create custom mounting brackets and cutting the fenders to fit, greatly adding to the cost and shortening the life of the fenders.

For colder weather rides, you'll want a thicker, thermal riding jacket. With a similar cut to the windbreaker, this is intended to be worn throughout your entire ride. It comes equipped with back pockets similar to those on your jersey, providing you with easy access to your food and other supplies on a cold day without having to remove a layer. Many of these also come with a bit of wind protection (especially over the chest) and light water resistance, and they are usually the most breathable of all types of jackets. For the coldest days, it's great to layer one with your windbreaker or vest on top for extra protection.

Then came the rain. If you live in a climate that sees a lot of wet weather, a cycling rain jacket is a godsend. The rain jacket is heavier than a windbreaker (but has similar, element-blocking properties), and there are a few different types to try when you want to dodge raindrops. Which jacket is right for you will come down to how long and often you plan to ride in the rain, and how completely waterproof you need it to be. In general, the more waterproof the material, the less breathable (and more sweat generating) it is.

For racers or serious fitness cyclists, there are rain jackets that are form-fitting yet and can pack down almost as small as a windbreaker. These can be anything from a bit of inexpensive plastic to high-tech, semi-breathable materials that are still mostly or entirely waterproof. For commuters and cycle tourists, there is a more heavy-duty-style rain protection. Although this type of coat won't fit in a pocket and has a much less aerodynamic fit, it's intended to be worn for your entire ride over other layers. It's waterproof yet breathable due to both materials and venting in the armpits, back, and/or sides to make it more comfortable to wear for long periods of time, and help you not end up soaked from sweat at the end of your ride.

Arm, Leg, and Knee Warmers

"Warmers" are one of the most brilliant pieces of clothing ever invented, so much so that other sport industries have stolen the idea and run with it themselves. They are small sleeves designed to fit over specific parts of your body to extend your clothing—turning short-sleeved jerseys into long-sleeved jerseys, bike shorts into three-quarter-leg or full-leg tights, and then back again as conditions warrant. Their genius lies in that they are easily removable for changing conditions effectively, making your summer riding gear double as fall, winter, or spring gear—and doubling your wardrobe.

For example, if you head out on a chilly spring morning ride, you might need your arm and knee warmers to keep the cold out, but as the day warms you can easily shed them and tuck them away in a pocket. In the winter, you might switch to a full-leg warmer for better coverage. They come in different weights of materials depending on your preferred style—many are made with wool or have fleece linings for maximum coziness and wicking.

Gloves

Cycling has what can look to the new rider like a somewhat frivolous accessory—fingerless gloves. This is what most riders often wear for a few really smart reasons. One, the gloves come with extra-thick material on the palms to protect your hands in case of an accident—because your natural first reaction will be to put your hands out in front of you. Without gloves, you can end up with scrapes on one of the most sensitive parts of your body.

Many cycling gloves also come with specific padding to relieve pressure on the nerves in your wrists and hands. Hours of resting on the bars and absorbing road vibration can create numbness or, worse yet, pain in your hands and fingers. This little bit of selectively placed padding can make a huge difference in comfort.

There are, of course, full-fingered gloves for warmth and protection in the winter. Typically what makes these special is the same padding with additional thermal material for warmth, some added wind or water repellency, plus reflective material (because winter rides are often in less than optimal lighting conditions).

Head Gear

There are lots of things besides helmets to protect your head—not to mention your ears and eyes. To absorb sweat and give you minimal

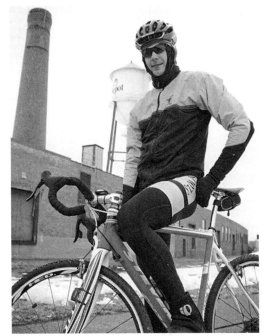

Whether you run hot or cool, you have lots of options for layering up when the weather turns foul.

eye protection from the sun, there are small, traditional cycling caps that fit under your helmet. Some people don't like having a visor on a hat, or prefer to have the visor attached to their helmet but still want perspiration absorption. A bandanna or do-rag fits nicely under the helmet.

In the winter, hats vary from tight skullcaps to caps with visors and special earflaps built in. Cold-weather caps are made almost exclusively out of polyester or merino wool. You can also buy a special earflapped headband that fits over your summer cycling cap if you find that winter caps are too big or bulky.

For the coldest, most extreme weather conditions, which, thankfully, many of us will never ride in, balaclavas (the ski masks made infamous by bank robbers) are one option. Another option is a neck warmer (a.k.a. neck gaiter or winter collar) that will block the cold air from channeling down the front of your coat and into your core. These are also available in very lightweight, ultra-wicking UV blocking materials if you ride in places with high elevation and lots of sun, and don't want to constantly slather on sunscreen.

No matter what time of year, keeping your eyes protected is a great idea. We're used to thinking of eye protection in terms of the sun, but on the road you'll be subjected to the occasional flying rock, road dust, low branch, or swarm of bugs, and it doesn't take much to cause a serious injury that could easily be avoided with riding glasses. That lovely breeze on your face will be a constant as well, and glasses are great to help your eyes from tearing up.

Shoe Covers

You can just wear thicker socks—but only to a point. Because of the narrow fit of cycling shoes, you can't bulk up too much or you'll actually make your feet colder faster by cutting off the circulation you need to bring that warm blood through. This is why these fabric covers that slide over your shoes are lovely little additions that keep your toes nice and toasty in colder weather. They come in two lengths—simple toe covers and full booties that come with a small cutout for clipless pedal cleats. Much like jackets, the booties come in different fabric weights and levels of protection depending on weather conditions. The thicker and more waterproof they are, the less they are able to let your feet breathe.

Sunscreen and Windscreens

A word about protecting your skin. As we mentioned in both the arm/leg/knee warmer and headgear sections, in recent years there have been many products created to protect us from the sun. As the ozone layer depletes and UV rays become more insidious, protecting our skin from cancer-causing damage is no longer an option, but a must. Cyclists spend hours at a time in the sun, so make sure exposed skin—especially your neck (which because of your riding position gets the most exposure)—is coated in sunscreen. If you're out for more than 2 hours, bring a small tube to reapply.

Of course, fabric sunscreens are more effective and not only block the sun's powerful rays but also eliminate the need to slather yourself in creams. They also give you added protection from the hydration-sucking wind.

CHAPTER 18

The Things They Carried: What to Bring on Your Ride

THERE IS THE GEAR YOU WEAR, AND THEN THERE IS THE GEAR you want to have installed on your bike or carry with you in your pockets. Riders' gear can vary from ultra-light to the kitchen sink depending on their temperament and the type of riding they like to do.

Saddlebags

Let's start with the basics—the kinds of compartments you want to carry things in. The average road cyclist—no matter what type—has at least a saddlebag. This is a small bag (though they come in slightly larger sizes, too) that tucks under the back

Bringing Up the Rear: Your Saddle Bag

THIS IS THE HOLY GRAIL OF A cyclist's carrying devices. The bigger your saddle bag is, the farther you can go. Whether you ride minimalist or with everything but the kitchen sink, there's no shame in taking a page from the Boy Scouts: "Be prepared"!

Level I, Weight Weenie: You want the smallest, lightest, most compact bag possible.

Carry:
- A tire lever (or two)
- Tube—out of box and tightly wrapped in plastic wrap for ultimate shrinkage
- Patch, glue, and emery cloth (essentially a patch kit without the box)
- Cash (for food, bus fare, or as an emergency tire boot to keep the tube from pushing out of larger holes or gashes in your tire)
- CO_2 and inflator
- ID/insurance card/debit card (Note: Debit card does not work as a replacement for cash in a tire boot.)

Level II, Easy Rider: You ride solo a lot and are wary of getting stranded.

Add:
- Duct tape (1 foot wrapped around a small piece of cardboard)
- Tire boot (reinforced piece of rubber to protect your tube from large gashes in your tire)
- 1–2 more tire levers
- Small multitool
- Presta-to-Schrader valve adapter
- Hand pump (may be carried on bike or in pocket)

Level III, Not Counting Grams: You'd rather be safe than sorry.

Add:
- Extra tube
- Emergency energy gel or bar
- A master link or replacement pin for chain repair
- Chain breaker
- Go to a bigger multitool with all the works.

Level IV, Going the Distance: You're in it for the long haul.

You have a really long commute or are touring. You're not afraid of the weight, but wary of the cold dark rain. Your small seat pack has morphed into a carrier clamped to the seatpost. You are just short of actually having a rack installed on your bike.

Add:
- Zip ties
- Lights
- Lightweight jacket/extra clothes
- Emergency spoke replacement
- More extra food
- Spare batteries
- 4-inch crescent wrench
- Anything else you don't think you can live without

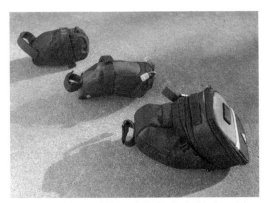

Whether you're going light or throwing in the kitchen sink, there's a saddle bag for you.

end of your saddle. It's intended to carry your flat repair items, a few small tools, and maybe emergency money or energy gel (for more on what to carry, see "Bringing Up the Rear" at left). It's limited in space, so it can really just hold the basics that you'll need for every ride but don't want to have to pack each time. It usually will live under the saddle on your bike.

Bento Bags

If you want to have more food or a wallet that won't fit into your jersey pocket, there are "bento" bags, which rest in front of you on the top tube of the bike for easy access while pedaling. They're usually the size of a very large wallet and can carry a few extra snack bars, some cash, or your sunscreen—anything you want close at hand.

Handlebar Bags

For cycle-tourists who need to carry everything they need for day of riding and sightseeing, there are large bags that hang off the front of the handlebars that can hold a great deal—all of the stuff you can put in a bento bag, times 10. A camera, food, your wallet, extra clothing— really quite a bit can fit inside. Some have a specially designed window so you can have your route map for the day sitting where you can see it while riding and keeping it safe from sudden downpours. The downfall of these bags is that they catch a lot of wind, though for the cycle-tourist who is weighed down with gear, this usually isn't an issue.

Panniers

Finally, there are panniers, which are very large bags that hook onto a mounted rack. They are purchased in pairs, because they are designed to go on both sides of your rack and can hold everything from tents and food to laptops and clothes. So of course, before you get them you have to buy and install a rack, which most road bikes (other than touring and some cross-discipline bikes) will not be designed to accommodate because they are built for speed over carrying capacity. The average road bike is like a sports car (sleek and aerodynamic), while the touring bike is more of the minivan or pickup truck. They can both get you there, but the trip will be significantly different. If you're planning on carrying panniers or any bag that mounts to a rack, make sure you buy a bicycle that can take one first.

There are racks and panniers designed specifically for the front or rear of the bike. If using racks, most riders start out with a rear only since weight in the front makes the handlebars harder to control. The beauty of pannier design is that it allows your extra weight to sit low (as opposed to up high on top of a rack or on your back), keeping your center of gravity closer to the ground and your ride much more stable. The downside to saddlebags is, of course, that you lose a great deal of aerodynamics. For some riders—like cycle-tourists or commuters—this will be an acceptable compromise to carry your gear.

Pump vs. CO$_2$

No matter what you carry in your saddlebag, at minimum you'll need a new tube, some tire levers, and an inflation device. At home you'll use a floor pump, but when it comes to airing up your tires on the road, it really comes down to two choices: a hand pump or CO$_2$.

Hand Pumps

These are a great option for almost any ride because of their dependability. You can use them to find the hole in your tube, refill your tire after a flat, and for a quick top-off on the road. The most minimal are usually the smallest, but the smaller the pump, the more strokes (and therefore time and effort) it will take to fill up your tire. A pump with a small hose attachment is recommended to make it easier to use without damaging the valve stem on the tube. Some larger and more deluxe hand pumps even convert into miniature floor pumps with fold-out footrests and handles to make using them a breeze. Most hand pumps also come with mounts to attach to your bike, but it's also common for riders to slide the pump into their jersey pockets.

Frame Pumps

These are directly related to the hand pump. They lack a hose and some other features, but have a large air chamber that can make filling your tire faster. They use a spring system to compress the pump between the tubes of your frame so you don't need a special mount. However, many modern carbon fiber or aluminum frames have odd-shaped tubing that makes it hard for these pumps to fit properly.

CO$_2$

If time is of the essence (like during a race or on a group ride where people are waiting for you), CO$_2$ may be a better choice. Instead of having to spend 3 minutes or more filling your tire after you've replaced the tube, you can reinflate in a matter of seconds. The CO$_2$ cartridge is a thumb-sized metal canister with pressurized carbon dioxide that comes in two sizes—12 or 16 gauge—the larger of which is for road bike tires. You'll also need a special inflator to break the seal—the best of which have a lever to allow you to control how quickly and how much air goes into your tire.

The plus side is the speed of inflation, but CO_2 has its downside, too. If you have more than one flat—or accidentally release the CO_2 trying to fill your tire—you've lost one of your chances to repair the flat and get home. Because of the weight of the cartridges, you don't save grams. You'll also be carrying the empty metal canisters home with you after you've used them. An important note: CO_2 won't keep your tire inflated longer than overnight. Plan on refilling it with good old-fashioned air from your floor pump the next morning if you find it's a little low.

Some people find that carrying both a pump and CO_2 is the best solution. That way you have speed when you want it, but a backup if you need it. With either choice, make sure you practice using it once or twice before you hit the road so when the time comes, you don't have to figure out how the thing works.

Computers

We have them at home. We have them on our phones. We use them as our TVs. It only makes sense that our bicycles would have them, too, right? Some riders just want to ride, enjoy the scenery, and use the time on their bikes to unplug from technology. For others, computers can be an invaluable training tool to keep track of changes from one ride to the next or follow cue sheets for turns when touring or on a club ride, or as motivation to meet certain goals or markers. The bottom line is, you don't need a computer to enjoy riding, but if you think it would be a good fit for you, there are many to choose from.

All computers use a magnet attached to the spokes of your wheel and a sensor attached to the fork to collect information with each rotation of the wheel. The more basic and inexpensive computers have a long wire running from the fork reader to carry the information to the display on your handlebars ($15–$50). On the more deluxe models ($50–$90), the information is passed wirelessly and more functions are offered. On the most high-end models ($150+), the computer reader battery is generally rechargeable and there are ways to take the information gathered and upload it to your computer or phone to track your numbers.

Basic Functions
(Found on All Computers)

DISTANCE: Bicycle computers began as a simple odometer to track mileage on your rides. They still do, but now they also offer many more options specific to cycling needs. This includes a function that will let you track the distance of your current ride separately from the total mileage you've ridden with the computer (odometer).

SPEED: This can include your current speed (how fast you're going), your average speed (how fast you go over your whole ride), or your maximum speed (how fast you bombed down the hill).

TIME: Hey, who wears a watch these days? These functions include a clock (so you don't have to reach for your phone while riding) and also tracking total ride time.

WHEEL-SIZE SETTINGS: Since different-sized tires and wheels will change how far your wheel rolls on each rotation, most computers have codes to easily input the size you have on your bike.

Advanced Functions (Found on $40–$90 Wired and Wireless Models)

DUAL BIKE MEMORY: Allows you to use the computer on different bikes with different wheels and still get an accurate reading.

TEMPERATURE: So you can see how hard you had to work in the heat.

STOPWATCH: For interval training or if you are doing laps within one ride.

AUTO START/STOP: This allows your computer to stop tracking when you're stopped at lights or for a snack break so you have a separate recording of your moving time.

SLEEP MODE: Automatically powers down to help conserve your battery if you're stopped for more than a few minutes. Will "awaken" where you left off on your ride when you turn it back on.

ALTITUDE: This tracks how high and low you have hit on your ride and, more importantly, the total amount you climbed.

Advanced Functions (Found on Computers $150+)

CADENCE: This tracks how fast you're pedaling by counting the rpms (revolutions per minute) your pedals make. This is a good feature if you want to practice spinning more—which makes you both faster and more efficient. This also requires another magnet that attaches to your crank arm and another sensor attached to your frame.

HEART RATE MONITOR: One way to track how hard you're working is by measuring your heart rate. This can be very helpful if you are training for a race or event and want to do very specific workouts.

GPS: Computers with GPS allow you to track distance even without the traditional wheel sensor. The largest-screened and high-end devices even come with street maps, topography, and more.

UPLOADING DATA: This allows you to keep track of your numbers (distance, speed, heart rate, etc.) so you can use them for comparison and graph how your ride or race went. It also will keep track of your route, so you can always revisit a ride and see how you got there.

Phone Applications

If you're interested in keeping track of your rides—speed, distance, routes, elevation, and time—but don't want to buy a computer, there are now apps that allow you to do all of the above by making use of the GPS in your phone. Usually, they also have a social networking aspect that allows you to compare your ride times with friends or meet new people that you might want to ride with.

Like any app, the downside is that they are a huge battery suck, so if you ride a lot, you'll need a booster for your phone so it doesn't run out of juice. The upside is that the high-end computers with the "upload" function allow you to upload this same information into these apps on your home computer.

Either way, this can be a great way to find new routes, make ride buddies, and compete with local riders without having to race. All of which make them extremely valuable and, for some, extra fun.

Mirrors

You can attach a mirror to your helmet or to your handlebars if you feel it will help to keep you more aware of your surroundings or if you have a hard time looking over your shoulder due to some kind of physical limitation. The handlebar mirrors are a little tougher to see clearly because they pick up all the road vibration, so many prefer the helmet type.

Many riders prefer not to use mirrors at all because they find them either distracting or, in the case of the helmet mount, they may block some of the rider's forward field of vision.

CHAPTER 19

Let's Get Visible

LIKE MOTORCYCLES OR PEDESTRIANS, CYCLISTS ARE BUT A blip on the radar of most motor vehicle drivers. This is why making sure you can be seen can save your life. Contrary to how the media portrays cyclists, most of them are also drivers themselves. As you begin your journey on the bike, you'll likely start to pay more attention to cyclists when you're driving a car, noticing which of them are easy to spot on the road and which aren't. Then you can follow the lead of the notice-able ones. As far as gear goes, this is just one aspect of the new pieces you'll already be investing in. Here are some tips on how to help you stand out in the peripheral vision of drivers.

Keep Your Clothing Bright

This is a challenge for many cyclists because bright clothing is harder to keep clean of road grit and accidental brushes with bicycle grease. Invest in some good stain lifter and keep your colors bold.

Look for Reflective Accents in Clothing

In this high-tech world, there are many ways to make fabrics more reflective, from bits of coating to piping along the seams. Look for clothes that place strategic reflec-tive fabrics or coatings in places where cars will throw their headlights—particularly the sides and back. Some gloves have reflective bits to help hand signals light up. Rain jackets in particular should have good bits of reflection since in most states, cars are required to drive with their lights on in the rain.

Look for Reflective Accents in Your Bicycle's Gear—or Add Some On

These days, everything from fenders to saddlebags to helmets come with reflective surfaces. If they don't or if you'd like to add more, there are options from simple reflective tape to fun, bicycle-centric decorative reflective stickers to make both your bike and your personality shine.

Lights Are the Best (and Sometimes Mandatory)

If you're riding at night, most municipalities in the United States have laws requiring cyclists to have lights to help with visibility. But cover of darkness isn't the only place they come in handy. Rain makes most vehicles lose a good percentage of their clear sight lines. Everyone can be enveloped on a foggy day. In general, you'll want at least one front and rear light, and if you ride where it's particularly dangerous, you might want a few of each—especially in the rear since you'll be riding with the flow of traffic and the most common accidents either come from behind or from someone passing you then making a right-hand turn in front of you.

Lights vary from inexpensive, non-rechargeable battery-powered LEDs to mid-range USB rechargeable lights you can conveniently plug into your computer to motorcycle-strength lights with large, heavy batteries—these last are a big investment but they both help you be seen and also light up the road enough that it's almost as bright as riding during the day. How much you want to invest in your light should be proportional to how much riding you do in the early morning or late evening hours.

PART VI

ROAD RIDING SKILLS: BEING ONE WITH THE BIKE

You've got your bicycle, you've got the gear, so you're ready to roll, right? Well . . . maybe. To be safe and have fun on the bike, you want to be in command under all circumstances—and good leadership starts with finding your little "home away from home" in the saddle. You'll want to get to know your body's strengths, weaknesses, and preferences to use all of them to your advantage. The best captains are also the coolest and calmest. No one feels safe under a panicky, unstable leader, so being relaxed on the bike is an essential component of riding well.

We'll get you familiar with which of your feet is your "power pedal" and which is your balance leg. Like being right- or left-handed, most of us are right- or left-footed. Each of us favors one side for power and the other for stability, so deciphering which foot will lead gives you more control in cornering, climbing, turning—really everything that involves balance, strength, and shifting weight distribution on the bike.

There are at least four different riding positions on the bike, each optimizing changes in terrain, what you want to accomplish, and how your body is feeling. Once you settle into each of these, your bike and your body will be more confident, allowing you to be a smoother rider. This will also let you concentrate on the job at hand—whether that's better climbing or descending, or paying attention to the road and the riders around you.

Shifting is its own mystery for most riders—even those who have been on the bike a while. Even when you've figured out how to get the gears to switch, it's another matter to know when to change them to easier or harder gears to optimize your strength and endurance—not to mention to keep from busting a lung getting to the top.

Whether you're sharing the road with your fellow riders, motor vehicles, or pedestrians, predictability is key to being a good neighbor. Within that concept is being an ambassador of the rules of the road—obeying all traffic controls, using hand signals, and being courteous to pedestrians. It means not only having a steady, even-keeled ride, but also communicating all the time. Whether that's through using hand signals, checking over your shoulder, or even using your voice, you want to be clear about where you are, where you're going, and any obstructions that might lie ahead. Each group ride—whether it's 2 people or 200—will change depending on the group you're riding with. As a good rider, you'll have to be flexible to the needs of the group—and on some days that might even mean you decide to ride alone.

CHAPTER 20

Everything in Balance: Beginning Riding Position

WHETHER IT WAS THE KARATE KID OR LUKE SKYWALKER, THE wise men of 1980s movies learned that to do anything well, you have to start from the basics. "Wax on, wax off" and "feel the force" were the building blocks—without them, your opponent would handily beat you down.

First off, remember that the bike is on your side—although gravity may be your foe, your bicycle is not. Its spinning wheels naturally create a gyroscopic effect due to their centrifugal force. This effect makes it extremely difficult to tip over while in motion. So the first key to balance is having enough momentum to keep upright. As long as you're moving around 5 to 6 miles per hour (which is a very average walking pace), your bike will keep moving forward, usually in a straight line.

When it comes to balance, three is a magic number for points of contact with the bike. Your body contacts the bike at the handlebars, the seat, and the pedals. Of these, the handlebars and pedals are the most important part for staying balanced and in control of your bike—which is why it's easier to stand up and pedal than to ride with no hands. Your handlebars are a no-brainer because they obviously are used to steer. The body weight resting on your pedals through your feet is just as important though, because that downward pressure—especially when it's applied evenly—will also help to keep your equilibrium.

Just like in the movies where the heroes spend countless, mindless hours getting the basics down pat before they move on, you'll want to practice these skills often if you're just learning to get comfortable with a road bike. If you're very new to riding, practice in a parking lot or on a bike path. Like the stars that save the day, you'll want the basics to become second nature before you test them on the road—where traffic, other riders, and unforeseen obstacles are added into the mix.

A word of support for the novice road rider: If you have never captained a road bike, your first rides may feel as if your body is being thrown unnaturally, dangerously far forward. Because your whole torso is lower to the ground, it can seem as if you may go over the bars at any second and that your teeth are in danger of being rearranged by pavement. Stay relaxed and continue to practice in low-traffic areas. In short time, your fight-or-flight reptilian brain will learn this position is as comfortable and as safe as any other—because it is. Have patience if it doesn't seem natural on day one. Like anything new, time and practice will eventually make it seem second nature.

How your body sits on your bike will never be static. Cyclists shift their weight around as the road beneath them changes. Whether climbing a hill, descending, shifting, or experiencing bumps, moving your center of gravity will help the bike work to your advantage.

Wherever you're in contact with the bike, you are the suspension system. Think of how badly your car would drive if you didn't have shocks and every little bump translated directly into the steering wheel. Yikes. In the case of the bike, you have natural absorbers built into your body—your shoulders, neck, hands, wrists, elbows, knees, ankles, and feet. That's a lot of vibration dampening, but it works only if you stay *relaxed*. This is the key to hours of enjoyable, safe riding.

Strangely enough, this starts not at any of those joints, but in your diaphragm (the big muscle below your lungs that controls your breath). Make sure you're taking full, deep, steady breaths—especially if you're in a situation that makes you nervous or excited (like a sprint in a race). The more you clench up, the faster you'll lose control. Also practice letting go of tension in your arms, shoulders, and neck. Keep all of your joints soft and slightly bent. The more rubbery and loose they are, the quicker they'll be able to respond to changes in the road and the less fatigued you'll become. Staying relaxed saves energy and keeps you in the best control possible.

NEUTRAL POSITION: This is where the bike is

designed to be ridden most of the time—on flat or gently rolling ground. Your hand position will generally be on top of the hoods where you have access to the brakes and shifters. If the bike is properly fit, you should be able to freely turn your head and neck to look around, should not have too much pressure on your hands, and should feel comfortable sitting for extended periods of time. If you're riding for long stretches where you don't foresee shifting or stopping (and you're confident that you can move your hands quickly to the hoods to access the brake levers in an emergency) you can also switch your hands to the top of the bars, closer to your body. This will allow you to take some weight off of them and change your back and neck position slightly.

In either of those hand positions, you'll want to keep your bottom square on the saddle when riding in neutral. If you took a snapshot of your body from the side while riding, your torso and arms should make an almost perfect 45-degree angle. As mentioned before, your feet should be taking a good portion of your body weight into the pedals, so your saddle isn't overloaded.

Having a seat position that is too low can cause serious problems for your knees, hips, back, and, most critically, your booty. Low saddle height causes the weight to be unevenly distributed into your sit bones and the soft tissue between them. This can cause discomfort quickly—even on a seat that fits you properly.

Your spine should be straight, keeping your back, neck, and head in alignment. Keep your

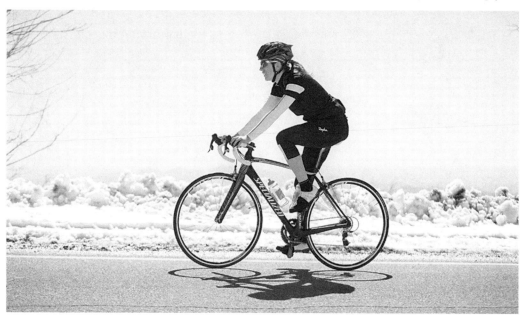

Neutral position is relaxed and centered.

shoulders broad and away from your ears, and your chest forward. This allows your airways to remain open and makes it easier to breath. Keeping good posture will also prevent the cyclist "hunch" that plagues riders, causing neck, shoulder, and back pain. If you feel as if you can't easily do this without straining, the bike may need a professional fit.

DROPPED POSITION: When you need to lower your torso or center of gravity, the C-shaped lower portion of your handlebars—called the "drops"—is there for you. This position is most often used when descending, especially down long, steep inclines. Your torso will be bent more forward from the hips and your wrists will torque up a bit so you can readily reach the brake levers.

Riding in the drops makes it slightly harder to shift, but makes huge gains in braking ability—especially helpful on extended downhills—because you have a closer reach to the brake lever for both a quicker reaction time and the leverage to make a more powerful stop. This seems as if it would increase the pressure on your hands, and while it does, you'll also be taking most of your weight into your feet because you're coasting downhill.

When you shift to this position for descending, you'll also make a slight shift of your weight back off your seat. Note that while you're taking your bottom off the saddle, you're not raising it up much, but bringing it backward toward the rear wheel to give you more traction. Your body will naturally shift forward on downhills, and

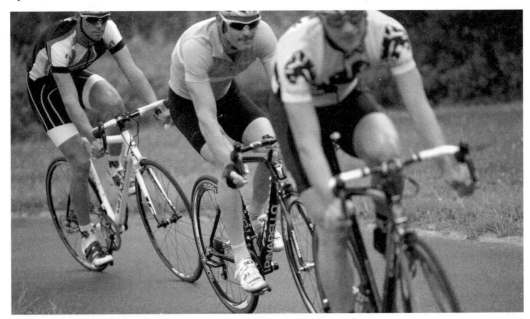

The dropped position helps keep you steady on descents and gives you power in sprints.

this position allows you to push the weight back a bit to counterbalance.

By bringing your hands lower on the bars, your torso also shifts closer to the ground. This is good, because a lower center of gravity will make it much easier to balance and stay in control. If you try to remain in neutral position on steep descents, it will be harder to brake and your high center of gravity will make you feel wobbly and less stable. Again, your spine should be as straight as possible.

This same principle is applied to cornering. The shift in weight distribution helps you stay stable and in good contact with the ground.

Because riding in the drops is so much more aerodynamic, it is also a great choice for battling headwinds. Taking your torso and face out of the wind can add a few miles per hour to your speed. Pedaling in the drops changes which muscle groups are called on for power. When trying to beat a headwind, staying seated in the saddle will shift the workload to your glutes. Especially if you've been on the road for a few hours, this shift can give your other muscle groups a much-needed break.

Finally, if you're a racer, the drops are where you'll head for your big sprints. This time, instead of grabbing the bars near the curve and close to the brakes, you'll hold the flat part close to the bars' ends. Raising your back and hips straight out of the saddle, you can push and pull on the bars for the ultimate leverage to help your legs pump. For anyone who's watched a pro bike race, this is a somewhat difficult maneuver because it's easy in this position to look straight down at the road and forget to watch where you're going. Also, torquing the bars for force makes it harder to steer straight. Don't try this for the first time in a race situation—get plenty of practice in first.

STANDING POSITION: As you spend more time in the saddle and find your comfort zones, this is a more intermediate maneuver. Standing on the pedals calls for using yet another muscle group, so most riders find it difficult to do for longer than 30-second to 1-minute intervals

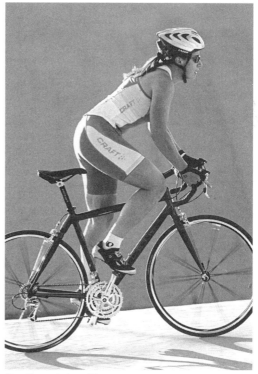

Standing up helps with power.

before their legs fatigue too much to continue. Most often, cyclists stand on the pedals to climb but also use the move to give their muscles and soft tissues a break.

To stand, place your hands on the hoods in your neutral riding position. As you rise up, your weight will naturally shift a bit forward, which will cause your bike to lurch. Keep your arms relaxed so you can easily make this transition without swerving the handlebars. Also note that for a split second your speed will slow during this transition. If another rider is close behind you, give them a little warning first.

With your torso slightly bent forward, keep your hips (which essentially are your center of gravity) still, mostly centered above and just in front of the nose of the saddle. It should almost look like you're on an elliptical machine—the legs doing almost all the movement with very still hips, arms, and torso. You may use your arms for some side-to-side torque, but the movement is happening in the bike, not in your body. Though the bike may be tilting from one side to another, it should still be traveling in a perfectly straight line. This is how you conserve the most energy.

CHAPTER 21

Just Riding Along: Starting, Stopping, and Everything Between

AT ITS MOST BASIC, THE BIKE IS DESIGNED TO DO TWO THINGS: go and stop. One will get you rolling, the other will save your life. Both are pretty important to having a good time on the road. There are many little pieces involved in getting going, staying rolling, and using your bike to the best of your body's ability.

From pushing off to get started to clipping in and out of your pedals to holding your line before you stop and clip out, there are many tips and tricks that can make being on your bike more enjoyable. We'll get you up to speed and riding like a pro in no time.

Shifting is a mystery to most people, something riders either just kind of "feel" their way through, or try not to do at all. This is bad for you and your bike, so it's important to break down what your shifting does and how to best use it to your advantage. Cadence is how fast your pedals rotate—which is directly related to what gear you've shifted into. Because the terrain beneath you is ever changing, you'll be shifting so your pedals can remain at the same tempo no matter what the circumstances.

To most new riders, the assumption is that turning a corner is like driving a car—you turn the wheels. When you're on a two-wheeled vehicle, everything changes. Your steering comes from your weight distribution, body placement, and leaning your bike. A similar approach will be applied to climbing and descending.

In no time at all, these will become second nature to you, and these skills will give you a huge advantage over riders who may have inadvertently picked up bad form when learning, then turned it into a bad habit. These cyclists have to work harder later to make their technique smooth, while you'll make owning the ribbon of road before you look effortless.

Starting and Stopping

Much as it is with our hands, most of us have one foot that is dominant. We'll call this the power leg. It often will follow your handedness. The other is your helper, the balance leg. Although it has less power, it has the more important job—to keep you stable when you're stopped on the bike. To figure out which is which, balance on each leg while holding the

other off the ground. Generally, your dominant side will not be as stable as your balance side.

To mount, grab the hoods of the handlebars and hold the brakes. This will keep the bike stable while you move around on it. Stand on your balance side about a foot away from the bicycle with your body facing forward. Lean the bike toward you (which will naturally lower the seat) and swing your power leg over the back end of the saddle from the rear of the bike, landing your dominant foot on the opposite side pedal. You should end up with your power foot solidly on the pedal (if you're riding clipless, you should be clipped into the pedal) with the saddle resting against the inner thigh of your balance leg, continuing to hold a firm grip on the brakes. You're almost ready to roll.

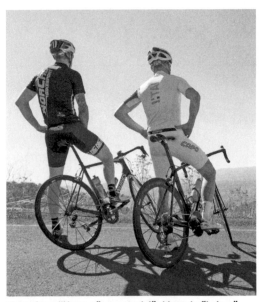

Most of us will have a "power pedal" side and a "helper" side for balance.

As we talked about in Chapter 20, which covered balance, the easiest way for the bike to stabilize is when it is rolling forward at 5 to 6 miles per hour (a walking pace). The quickest way to get it in motion is to put force into the pedal—and there you are with your dominant foot on the pedal, ready to go. You'll want your first pedal stroke to be as solid and strong as possible, so spin your dominant foot's pedal into a high, forward position

Clipping In and Out of Clipless Pedals

WHEN YOU BUY YOUR PEDALS, have the shop install them, then put your bike in one of their trainers and practice these motions over and over. It is easiest to clip in the pedal at the bottom of the stroke, closest to the ground at the 6 o'clock position. The pedal has a spring that, when you push down and forward firmly with the cleat that is bolted to the bottom of your shoe, opens slightly to allow your shoe to become attached.

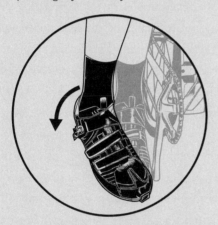
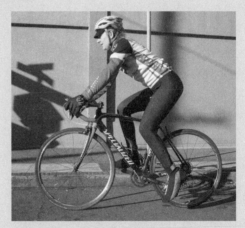

To release, keeping your feet level to the ground with your dominant foot forward in the 3 o'clock position, press down lightly while twisting your foot so your heel kicks out slightly away from the bike. It should not take much effort to do this. Many pedals have adjustable springs to make this motion easier. If you find this very difficult, have the shop adjust the spring tension until you're able to easily release your foot. Get used to releasing your balance foot first so when you come to stops you're ready to reach your leg out.

Practice in the trainer—20, 30, 50 times— until it feels somewhat natural. Then get ready to try it on the road. Always unclip your feet as you slow down but well before you're stopped. You can still rest your shoes on your pedals for stability, just don't have the cleats engaged. That way you're ready to put down your balance foot as soon as you come to a stop. Practice in quiet, low-traffic areas before you head out for a long ride.

(around 2 o'clock) so you'll be ready to push down. No matter where you stop, this is the easiest way to get started again with the least wobbling.

Simultaneously, gently push off once with your balance leg as you push down forcefully on your power pedal. This will give you the momentum you need to get the bike rolling forward and stable so you can find your second pedal with your balance foot (and, if necessary, get it clipped in). The number one place new riders struggle is giving the power pedal enough force to gain momentum. Don't be shy. Give it your all! Remember to also avoid looking down at your pedals. Your bike will always go where you look, so if you look down, your bike is likely to go down. Keep your eyes, chin, and neck upward, relaxed, and focused.

Holding Your Line

Holding your line is cycling's way of saying "Don't swerve around." As a good cycling ambassador, you want to be as predictable and in control as possible for the drivers and other cyclists around you.

The same basic principles of balance are put into place here. Make sure you've always got your three magic points of contact—handlebars, seat, and pedals. Losing your contact with the seat is like cutting off one of the legs of a three-legged stool. This is the reason why it's so much harder to hold your line when you're standing up on the pedals as opposed to in a neutral, seated position on the bike.

Stay as relaxed as possible. Most of the time you should be looking up and ahead, at least 20 feet in front of you. A general rule behind the physics of cycling is that your bike will go where you look. Want to avoid that stick in your path or that pothole? Look past it, and you'll steer *around* it instead of *at* it.

That being said, the ability to look around you—particularly to check over your left shoulder for traffic approaching from behind—without weaving the bike is a critical riding skill. Even if you use a mirror, you can't depend on it completely to let you know what's going on behind you. Practice turning your head while continuing to ride in a straight line. Don't hit the road for your first extended ride until you have thoroughly mastered this technique.

When you think you've mastered all these, practice them as slowly as possible. Because momentum keeps you upright and stable, the less speed you have, the harder it will be to ride in a straight line. The most skilled cyclist can look around, take one hand off the bars, stand up on the pedals, and more while holding the line at very low speeds. Practicing this can get you from novice to expert in no time.

Stopping

Just hit the brakes, right? Well, mostly. Most new riders think brakes keep their bikes in control—and while they do help, like most things in life, too much of a good thing can be bad for you. When you start riding, you might be tempted to either not go too fast (riding the brakes all the time) or, when confronted with a stressful scenario, slam on the brakes. Again, you need momentum for the bike to be balanced, so neither choice is great if you want to stay upright. Using too much of the brakes can actually make you fall. So when it comes to brakes, remember, temperance is your friend.

As you brake, your momentum forces most of your weight over the front wheel, making your front brake the more powerful of the two. However, if you use only the front, it can lock up and flip you over the handlebars. Your rear brake is strong, too, but it will never work very effectively because as you slow and your weight shifts forward, it causes the rear wheel to drag—creating a skid that can make you fishtail all over the road. Fun as a kid, but not so much in traffic.

Since the front brake has about 70 percent of your stopping power, but can send you flying, and the rear brake will make your tire drag and lose traction, the best solution is to use both brakes evenly. Like two best buddies, this technique makes them temper each other, bringing out their most powerful stopping power and your smoothest, safest braking.

As your weight is being thrown forward, it's good to push your body back a bit on the saddle as you slow down—and even farther in an

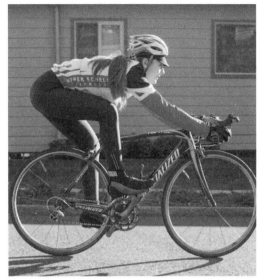

Pushing your weight back will help you keep traction during an emergency stop.

emergency stop. It will not only keep you from going over the bars, but will also help keep your rear wheel in traction and prevent skidding. Like a fire drill, you want to practice sudden, hard emergency braking so that it will become an automatic response in a high-pressure situation.

When the roads are wet, keep in mind it will take longer to stop. The traction between your pads and rims is greatly decreased because of the water coating them, so if you see a stop coming or are on a descent, apply the brakes lightly early on to clear the water from them, then brake harder. Even grabbing a handful of brake may not be enough to stop in the time you usually would. Plan far in advance for wet stops.

One-Handed Riding

THERE ARE MANY, MANY TIMES A RIDER will have to ride with one hand. This can be tricky because it affects your center of balance and how your weight is distributed. But it's critical to riding on the road because the only way we have to communicate with the world around us is hand gestures. If you can't confidently ride one-handed, you should not be riding with traffic.

As always, don't ever take one hand off the bars unless you know you can control the bike. You'll be losing the use of one brake, so take that into consideration before you move your hand from the bars. If you're riding a loaded touring bike, the extra weight will make this especially challenging.

The easiest way to ride one-handed is to place your hands on the top, flat part of the bar closest to you. This gives you better balance and control of the bike and allows you to shift your weight around more easily.

Single-Handed Skill Build

1. **Ride with your left hand hanging by your side.** This is the foundation. Using your left hand preps you to signal to cars and other riders.

2. **Ride with your left hand up and out, away from your body.** Riders have to signal to one another to avoid road hazards, which are commonly on the right since you'll be riding with traffic on the right side of the road.

3. **With your left hand off the bar, look left over your shoulder for approaching traffic or hazards without swerving.** It's commonly referred to as a "shoulder check," and you can't make a left turn or change lanes without this essential skill.

4. **Reach for your water bottle.** This shifts your weight in a way that's entirely different from the other one-handed skills. Practice first while coasting and work up to attempting it while pedaling. Since you need to drink every 10 to 15 minutes, this is a must.

5. **Reach into your rear jersey pockets.** It's not likely you're going to stop every time you need to eat. If you're in a group ride or race, there is little to no stopping for food breaks and you need to eat at least a few times every hour.

6. **Ride with one hand off the bar in different grip positions.** You won't always be on top of the bar. Get comfortable with moving around.

7. **Practice braking gently with your other hand.** This maneuver can throw your balance off but is essential if you need to stop suddenly.

Getting in Gear: Shifting, Spinning, and Cadence

Your gears are the most misunderstood and underappreciated part of your bicycle. They are your best pal, your dear friend, your savior on painful climbs and can make you a hero by helping you get the most out of what your body has to give.

The thing is, we humans are pretty much weaklings. Except for the extraordinary few, we can only run so fast and pedal so hard, the average among us capable of creating only a paltry amount of oomph. Although our horsepower is not all that great, we can take advantage of the little we have by putting the chain on the cog that best suits our strength and goals, which is a pretty darn cool solution. The derailleur's job is to move the chain onto each of those gears. Thank you, magical derailleurs! You control them by moving cables that run from your shifter levers to each derailleur (your bike has two, one for your front gears and one over your rear).

Your right shifter lever is in charge of the gears that are attached to your rear wheel. These are the baby steps that will help you make small shifting adjustments. Cyclists use this shifter more often—for example, every time you come to a stop and then as you begin rolling again. Sometimes you'll need a bigger jump in how hard or easy it is to pedal—like when you start to climb a hill. For big changes, you'll use your left shifter, which controls the chainrings (the big gear rings close to the pedals).

In both the front and rear, your cogs that are closest to the inside of the bike (toward the center of the wheel) are easier to pedal. Since their positions are matched, it is easy for you to keep the line of the chain as straight as possible from front to back. The chain doesn't work well and will wear out quickly if you ride it with the gears on a diagonal—called "cross-chaining"—so you want to avoid being in the hardest in front and the easiest in back, or vice versa. If you have only two chainrings up front, this is a combination you won't be able to completely avoid, but if you're on opposite sides of the gearring, that's a good sign when you need to make one of the bigger shifts in the front gears

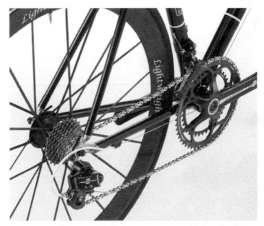

Your right shifter controls the rear gears, which make little changes; your left shifter controls the front chainrings, which make big jumps in how hard or easy it is to pedal.

Chainring, Cassette, Gear, or Cog?

EACH TOOTHED RING THAT THE CHAIN RIDES ON is commonly referred to either as a "cog" or a "gear"—different ways of saying the same thing. On the rear of the bike, the set of gears is called a cassette; in the front near the pedals, your gears are called chainrings.

to compensate.

Knowing when and how to shift seems like the most overwhelming part, but learning good shifting technique will increase the life of your chain, your cogs, your cables, and, most importantly, your body. Start by using only the rear shifter until you're totally comfortable and it seems second nature. While practicing with the right-hand shifter, leave your chain in the middle chainring in the front if you have three rings; or if you have just two in the front, keep the chain in the most inside (easier) gear.

"Spinning" Your Pedals

Turning your pedals in circles is easy, but *spinning* them in circles is not. What's the difference? The pedal makes a 360-degree rotation no matter where you put pressure on it. But making good use of the full 360 degrees is something that most of us have to learn how to do. If we look at the pedal stroke as a clock, it's intuitive to push down from about 2 o'clock to 5 o'clock on the downstroke. This is where you

have the most amount of leverage—and therefore power. (See the illustration in "Pedaling Like a Pro" on page 123.)

So why "waste" time and energy with the rest? Why not just use your best leverage? Using the full 12 hours of your pedaling clock shifts the bulk of the effort from your muscles to your heart and lungs. Your cardiovascular system is much more efficient than your muscles, which fill with lactic acid the more they are stressed, causing your muscles to carry less oxygen—this is the "burn" you sometimes feel when exercising—and making it increasingly it difficult for them to function properly. Also, utilizing your entire pedal stroke engages a wider variety muscle groups, further spreading the workload. Once you learn how to take advantage of the full 360 degrees, you'll be able to pedal faster and smoother and keep your legs from burning out too quickly.

Cadence

This fancy word really just means how fast you rotate the pedals, measured in revolutions per minute (rpm). A huge part of learning how to spin properly is training your body to pedal at a higher cadence.

When we learned to ride a bike for the first time, most likely it was on a single-speed bike. Pushing down hard on the pedals gave us speed and kept us balanced, both of which were pretty swell—especially if you were trying to race your friends around the block. So it became ingrained early that stomping on the pedals not only made us fast but also made us "fit." At the very least, you could *feel* how hard you were working—that must count for something!

Unfortunately, the way we learned to cycle as kids is actually very hard on our knees, backs, and leg muscles. So while it may have served you well in childhood, it's time to move on to a more sophisticated technique that will help you take full advantage of your legs, booty, heart, and lungs working together as a team. Though it's counterintuitive, this mostly involves keeping your feet moving in fast rotations that distribute your power as evenly as possible all the way around the pedal stroke. Usually this means pedaling much, much lighter and faster than most of us are used to.

Similar to weight lifting in the gym, you want to do either low reps and heavy weights (which will build your power and bulk you up) or high reps and lighter weights (which will tone your muscles and make you stronger overall), depending on what your goals are. As any good

trainer will tell you, if you try to pump big iron with a lot of reps with the idea that more of everything is better, you'll not only burn out quicker—you are also more likely to injure yourself. On bikes, always pushing big, difficult gears at a low cadence is the equivalent of going harder, not smarter, and often running head-first into injuries.

When starting to ride, most of us find that 50 to 70 rpm is where we are most comfortable, so your new goal is to keep your cadence between 90 and 110 rpm. The easiest way to find out how fast you're pedaling is to buy a computer that tells you your cadence. If a computer isn't in the budget, count how many times your right knee comes to the top of the pedal stroke for 30 seconds, then multiply that number by two.

Unless you're coming from a super-fit, athletic background, expect there to be a learning curve. This new style of pedaling may leave you feeling winded because your energy is being pulled from your not-yet-developed cardiovascular system. This is where a lot of new riders will give up on trying to get to a higher cadence. Don't despair! Although it may feel a little awkward and may strain your lungs at first, you will make significant improvements over short periods of time. Plus, it's much harder to correct bad form later.

As an exercise, practice pedaling much faster than normal for 5-minute intervals on a flat section of your ride. This will get your heart and lungs to shape up and make it easier to concentrate on your pedal stroke since it's only for a limited amount of time. As your body adjusts, increase the durations and the cadence until you're in the 90 to 110 rpm zone. Over a few months' time this will become second nature, your lungs will no longer burn, and when you want to go a little harder, you'll pedal faster instead of reaching for a higher gear that slows you and your legs down.

Pedaling Like a Pro

One tip of the pros is that keeping "light" on the pedals keeps them ready for anything their competitors throw at them. If they want to attack—or respond to a competitor's attack—they can quickly turn up the power and speed up their rpm without shifting. When they do choose to shift—say, to jump a gap or break away from the pack—it's nice, easy, and quiet because the tension on the chain is so low that the shift is whisper soft. Sometimes their competitors don't even know what hit them. Even if you never plan on racing, these techniques can help keep anyone safer on the road. It's important to be nimble moving with and through traffic. Sometimes you'll need a sudden burst of speed to make it through a yellow light or maneuver out of the way of a hazard. Being light is also being relaxed—an advantage in any situation.

Staying light on the pedals is all about spinning with smooth, evenly distributed power. There's an easy way to tell which part of the pedal stroke you're using. If your bum lifts slightly off the saddle when your cadence is high, it's because your legs are hammering downward—but neglecting the rest of the stroke. Your bottom will actually bounce a bit in the saddle at a higher cadence. This is referred to as "pedaling boxes"—the opposite of nice circles.

Starting with your right foot in the 2 o'clock position, control the power of your stroke so you don't just force it down. This will use a lot of the quads in the front and top of your leg. As you reach the bottom—the 4 o'clock to 7 o'clock position—imagine dragging the bottom of your shoe against the ground (as if you stepped in dog poop) or pushing yourself off on a cross-county ski or roller skate. Your foot should pull back, engaging your glute muscles.

At this point, your left foot is on the other side of the bike in the power position ready to push down, so your right foot will be tempted to slack off and take a break. Lifting up and over the back and top of the right pedal to complete your circle is the most important (and trickiest) part of the pedal stroke. Lift up and over through the 8 to 11 o'clock positions. Working this action above all others will take all the pressure off the down-stroke power in your other leg and allow your feet to move in beauti-

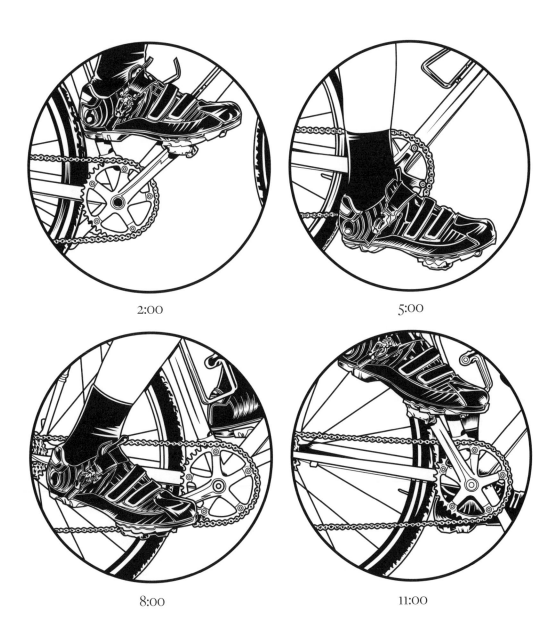

2:00

5:00

8:00

11:00

Having a clipless pedal allows you to use the full power of your entire pedal stroke.

ful, flowing circles. It's sometimes best to pull your foot up hard into the top of your shoe so it lifts slightly off the sole, then follow forward into the toe box over the top of your circle. This utilizes your calves and glutes, and feels a little bit like scrambling up a rocky slope.

You can concentrate on this positioning any-time, but pay special attention when you work on your cadence intervals and when climbing. These are the two times it's hardest to keep things together and flowing.

When to Shift

Cadence is all well and good, but to stay in a gear that's comfortable to spin in, you'll have to get familiar with when and how to shift. Antici-pation and timing are essential aspects of shift-ing smoothly. You can see when the road in front of you starts to pitch up or down, or that you're approaching a stop sign or red light. If you wait to shift until after your cadence has slowed, you'll lose your momentum—and with it some control of the bike.

The key to good shifting is consistency in pedaling. That does not mean staying in the same gear all the time, but instead staying in the same cadence zone as the road undulates and conditions change. In general, if the road goes uphill, you're in a headwind, or you're coming to a stop, you'll shift into lower gears to make it easier to pedal. If you're picking up speed from a stop, have a tailwind, or are head-ing downhill, you'll shift into higher gears.

The shifts you make with your right hand will compensate for the small changes in the road and wind. The large jumps you shift with your left hand deal with bigger changes—just like going up or down steep hills. As you get to know your bike and get more comfortable with cadence, you'll find yourself using your right shifter constantly throughout the ride and your left shifter less frequently. However, it's impor-tant to use both to your advantage, so find some times to play with both so you're comfort-able when the time comes to use them.

Downshifting

Downshifting means putting the bike into an easier gear—the gears closest to the inside of your bike. If your gears on a road bike were numbered, you'd be shifting into a one, two, or three in the rear and a one or two in the front. This is similar to a car with a stick shift, and the same basic principals are in place. Don't worry so much about numbers. Just remember: Keep-ing it low helps you go.

As we've discussed with cadence, the less tension on the chain, the better. So when you're approaching a stop, downshifting into a lower gear will set you up for a spinning start. Many of us tend to just stand up on the pedals to get moving, but this is very hard on the chain and gears, and also makes for a slower and more unstable start because it takes more time to give the bike momentum and get rolling up to full speed. Most of this shifting will likely take place with the rear gears unless you have to go up a hill immediately after the stop. Then you might want to make sure your chain is on the easiest gear on your front, too.

As the terrain tilts upward, it takes more power to get up the hill. To keep a fairly high cadence when climbing, you want to downshift before your pedals slow too much. Shift too late and your gears will loudly remind you that they prefer you make clean, smooth changes; shift too early and your legs will spin so fast that you will lose momentum. Start uphill in the easiest gear in the front, and then use the back gears to dial in the smaller adjustments of how fast you need to pedal. Realistically, no matter how strong we are, it's almost impossible to keep a cadence of 90 to 110 rpm going up a steep hill. Instead, aim for closer to 70 to 90 rpm.

When a headwind blasts you, it's tempting to grind your teeth, hunch over, and bear down on the pedals with all your might to fight back. Instead, downshift to a gear that makes it easy to keep spinning. It will sap less of your energy and keep you fresh to enjoy the inevitable tailwind when you head the other way. Best of all, once you're comfortable spinning, you'll find that you're able to keep a faster and more consistent speed in the face of the wind. It's no small feat to conquer Mother Nature!

Upshifting

Although most of the time the challenge will be to get your rpm high enough to spin properly, there's always a point of diminishing returns when your legs will be spinning too fast. If you don't have quite enough resistance on the pedals, you'll lose your momentum and, with it, your balance. That's when you'll want to upshift into a higher, harder gear.

Descending a hill is one of those times, as is when you've got a really strong tailwind or you're picking up speed from a stop. The biggest challenge of riding in a higher gear is looking ahead to know when you might need to downshift again. When you're cruising downhill in the blaze of a fantastic descent, it's easy to forget that the hill is going to bottom out. Make sure you downshift before the hill ends to keep you in a spinning gear for what comes next.

Climbing

Although there are mountain goats among us, most cyclists have to battle with their all-too-human nemesis: gravity. The laws of physics generally dictate that the tiniest among us will have the easiest time going up, followed by the strongest. These few individuals are blessed with a wonderful power-to-weight ratio—a scientific phrase meaning that they have less of a caboose to lug uphill or have a big, strong engine to push it. One thing to keep in mind is that no matter who you are, there's no sugar-coating the fact that hills hurt.

We all have it within our reach to temper that pain and master that climb by making the most of the gears our bike offers. The most efficient way to do this is to keep your butt in the saddle and keep your pedals spinning between 70 and 90 rpm. Don't avoid your lowest gears thinking it makes you some kind of hero. The pros will be the first to tell you that they use their lowest gears most of the time.

Stay relaxed. A death grip on the bars, grinding your teeth, and hammering the pedals is a huge waste of energy. When you chill out in the saddle, it's easier to take the fullest breaths possible—which will help deliver much-needed oxygen to your blood. Elbows and wrists should be loose on the bars.

Be patient. Your speed is going to slow quite a bit—possibly by almost half or more. Don't try to make up for it by madly attacking the hill. Pacing yourself is the key to keeping your heart rate and lactic acid in check so your legs don't blow up and you feel like you're killing yourself trying to get to the top. If you're in your lowest gear and you still can't make it to the top, pull over and briefly rest until your heart rate comes down, or walk. It's not cheating. It's not failing. It's using your brain to make the most of your body.

All cyclists, at some point in their cycling lives, have faced at least one hill they have had to walk—even the pros. A time will come when you'll build up the strength to conquer most hills. In the meantime, go easy on yourself and set smaller goals with the climbs around where you ride—like trying to make it up farther each attempt, or adding another hill to your route.

Shift your weight very slightly into the back of your saddle, which will give you the best leverage on your pedals. This also weights your rear wheel, giving it more traction. If the grade is very, very steep, you might have to shift the weight toward the nose of the saddle to keep the front wheel from popping up off the ground. In this case, remember that keeping your body relaxed is key.

As for climbing out of the saddle, it takes more energy to stand than to pedal seated because it shifts the work of your body from cardio to power. You'll literally be muscling up the hill. Most riders can climb like this only for a short time before they pop, so be strategic about when you stand. It's a perfect break for your seated muscles on a long ascent. It can also help you make it through an excessively steep section or, if you're racing, sprint away from the pack.

Before you stand up, upshift into one higher (harder) gear in the rear, which adds resistance—and therefore power and torque—as you push down. This will bring your average rpm down to around 60. Pull lightly on the handlebars for better leverage, moving the bike slightly from side to side beneath you. This will exaggerate the pushing down and lifting over of your pedal stroke more than your normal spin.

Descending: What Goes Up …

This is the good stuff. Coasting is a thing of beauty and the hard-earned break for your tired muscles. It's wind in your hair. It's the road unfolding in a ribbon before you, glimpsing breathtaking views with the world for the taking.

Newer riders tend to fall into two groups: those who'd like to descend faster than they're able, and those who are so terrified when the nose of their saddle points down that it feels less like a reward and more like a punishment. Although they may be worlds apart, both can rule gravity and make descending fast, safe, and fun.

Let's start off by busting some myths.

MYTH: Riding fast downhill is unsafe and out of control.

REALITY: Most pro riders and experienced cyclists can easily reach 30 to 60 miles per hour and not get into a wreck. Descending smoothly is all about staying within your boundaries—while letting the bike do the work.

MYTH: Using your brakes constantly the entire way down will guarantee that you're safe and in control.

REALITY: Riders who are tense and nervous are more likely to get in an accident because they're riding the brakes too hard. Great, easy descending comes with learning to depend on your eyes, breathing, and weight distribution much more than your brakes.

When we're put into a situation that makes us feel threatened or unsure, our breathing tends to become shallow, which in turns causes our whole bodies to tense up. Before you drop into a descent, take a few deep, even breaths. Do a quick body awareness check. Are your neck and shoulders tensed up to your ears? Do you have a death grip on the bars? If so, loosen up a bit. To be in control, you first have to let go of anxiety, which is why keeping your entire body relaxed—freeing up your shoulders, neck, elbows, wrists, hips, hands, knees, and ankles—is the key to focus and control.

Another common cause of accidents during descents is ego. Overconfidence leads to thinking today's the day to beat your friend down the hill or capture the next record. You may not be nervous dropping downhill, but it can be just as dangerous to be overly amped and raring to go. The key to great descending is an inner calm that allows you to absorb and react to the world around you in the moment.

Lowering your center of gravity keeps you grounded and stable, so getting your weight back and closer to the road is a plus. If the gradient is slight, most riders will choose to stay in the neutral position (hands on the top of the bars, grabbing the brake hoods) and shift their bottom back a bit on the seat. Once the road tilts down more aggressively, a high and tilted forward torso moves too much of your weight over the front wheel and you can topple over.

When the road drops deeply, reach your hands down to the forward part of the drops (the bottom curved part of the bar) where you can easily reach the brakes, then shift your weight back even farther on the saddle, adding traction to your rear wheel. If you're shy about facing downhills, this position can seem a bit intimidating at first. Gain confidence by practicing this dropping down and backward weight-shifting on smaller declines. After a few goes, you'll start to notice how much more con-

nected your wheels feel with the ground, and shifting to the drops will be a natural way to glide down the hill.

As for your feet, keep them level with each other as you coast and put a little pressure into them. This will help lift a little weight off your saddle and help the bike move smoothly beneath you, especially on rough pavement. Nervous riders tend to cling to their seat with their legs, which keeps them from being able to react instantaneously to changes in the road. This is another place to loosen up.

When you're traveling at higher speeds around bends, position the foot that's closest to the outside of the road down at the bottom of

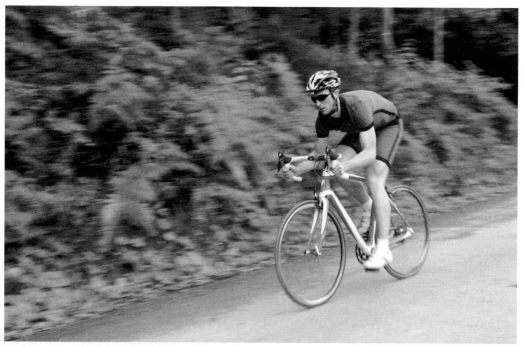

The key to a smooth descent is keeping your weight pushed back on the saddle and low in the drops.

your pedal stroke and press enough weight into it that you can lift a bit more from the saddle. As the bike leans beneath you, this will counterbalance your weight, keeping your body upright and helping your tires hold traction.

Of course, you should always be scanning ahead to watch where you're going, but when heading down hills, it's easy to look down just beyond your front wheel. Your bike is a trusty and faithful steed. It will go exactly where you look every time. If you peer only a few feet, you're going to be in trouble—especially on downhills. Keep your head up. When approaching curves, you need to turn your eyes, head, and neck to look around to the exit of the curve as opposed to in the middle of the bend.

Your brakes are there to be used *lightly*. Feathering them softly to scrub speed keeps the wheels from dangerously locking up in a skid. If you're intimidated by descents, you might be tempted to hold the brakes the entire way down. Bad idea. All that friction can heat up your rims, ultimately causing your tire to blow. Riding the brakes also makes it harder to keep your weight pushed back and your body relaxed, not to mention is a huge waste of your precious energy on what's supposed to be a rest period during the ride. Keep in mind, our friend momentum is on our side—but only if we keep it close. Ride too slow and you're more likely to swerve and wreck. That being said, if you're a speed demon, the judicious use of brakes is what creates an elegant and fast descent.

Always brake *before* corners—never in them when your tires are pushing the limits of contact and you're more likely to slide out. The curve will help your bicycle pick up speed so you'll exit at the same pace—or faster—than you went into it. Of course, that only applies when you actually make it through the turn. Don't be tempted to cross the mid-line into the oncoming traffic lane. A curve can be a life-altering mistake if you assume there isn't anyone coming around uphill on the other side.

If the road is wet, take extra care to go a little slower than you normally would. Water decreases traction and lifts the oils that vehicles shed to create a slick, lubricated surface. Even if it's not raining, damp or mossy roads should be ridden with caution.

Cornering

Carving a perfect turn is both sweet and satisfying. Most of us intuitively assume that steering comes by turning the handlebars. This is true at very slow speeds when you're lacking momentum, but most of the time you guide the bike around curves by leaning the bike in the direction of the turn. Luckily, a lot of the same concepts from descending are also applied here.

First, and we can't emphasize this enough—relax. Loose joints allow you to move around the bike easily and stay off the brakes. Next, look ahead, through, and around the turn. You'll be tempted to look straight into the corner of the turn. If you do, that's where you'll ride—likely right off the road. It's counterintuitive, but force yourself to look as far ahead down the road as possible by following one of the pavement markings until it disappears on the horizon. Sometimes this means that your head and eyes will be turned completely to one side—on sharp curves it can almost be to the point where you're actually looking over your shoulder. It may seem like you're not watching where you're going, but that's precisely what you're doing. By looking far ahead, your bike

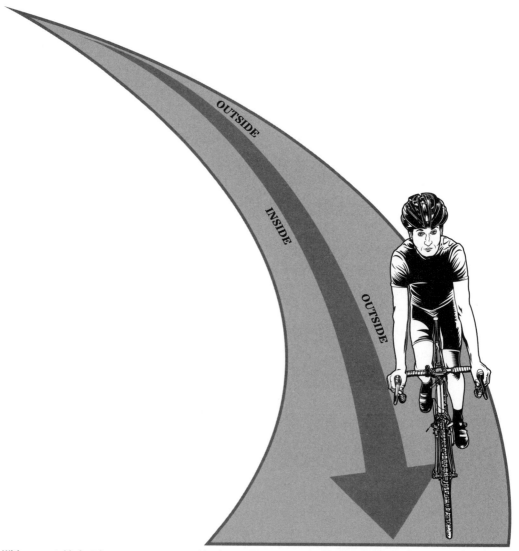

With your outside foot down, start your turns wide, then cut into the turn, and finish by exiting wide.

and body will naturally veer the right direction. If you're nervous that you'll miss a pothole or debris on the road in front of you, trust that your peripheral vision is strong enough that you'll notice if something comes up.

As you coast around the corner, make a wide arc with the bike. To do this, you'll be using the whole lane, so make sure traffic is clear behind you first. As you enter the turn, start with your bike close to outside of the curve. Riding into the turn, aim for the inside of the corner. As you exit, arc back into the outside of the turn. Out. In. Out.

One common mistake for new cyclists is to have the inside pedal down, which causes it to scrape against the ground. Position your feet so your inside pedal is all the way up and your pedal closest to the outside of the road is all the way down. This allows you to put some weight into it for added traction. By riding this way, you'll naturally angle the bike down toward the inside of the road. This tipping motion seems a little scary at first, but it takes advantage of the natural gravitational pull of the bike. If you try to fight this by keeping your bike upright, you'll lose traction and speed.

On the fast corners where you're holding a lot of speed, it's best to have your hands in the

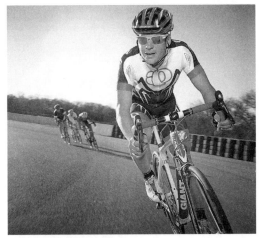

Safe turns come from weighting your outside foot for the best traction.

drops to lower your center of gravity and stabilize yourself as you cruise around the bend. Because the gravitational forces of riding through a curve will cause you to accelerate, always scrub most of your speed before entering the turn. Although it's almost impossible to not brake at all in a turn, you should already have slowed down enough that you only need to use the brakes barely, if at all. Braking hard in the turn is one of the worst things you can do. Quickly slowing changes your weight distribution and causes the bike to go from leaning and gripped to the road to upright, hard to control, and likely to skid out.

CHAPTER 22

Weather or Not: Battling the Elements

Wind

The sun is shining, the day looks perfect. Until you step outside and get blasted in the face with a gust of Mother Nature. Your first option is to check the weather and see what direction the wind is coming from. You might be able to adjust your route to best take advantage of the wind on the way home or stay out of it completely by keeping away from flat, open roads. Often, though, you don't have that choice.

Your body is essentially a big sail, and the bigger the load your bike has—say, if you're touring or commuting—the worse things will be. The trick is to do the best you can to minimize the effects of a head- or crosswind. This is why so much cycling-specific clothing is made to fit snugly and streamline your body as much as possible.

Ride with your hands in your drops and keep you head down as far as possible. Stay loose so you can quickly and easily react to sudden gusts. Forget your "normal" speed and shift into a low enough gear that you can pedal easily, and be prepared to keep shifting up and down as the wind changes. Keeping your cadence high and steady will make it much easier to endure the battle. Don't fight the breeze, embrace it.

If you're riding with others, take turns drafting. This means riding in a straight-line formation. The leader will create a wind break that the riders can take advantage of if they follow closely—within 2 to 3 inches—behind the lead rider's wheel. This allows some time to rest until their turn comes around to pull the group.

As soon as you turn around, your nemesis will become your best friend—the tailwind. While the wind can be cruel, it can also be generous. Learn to love both sides and your rides will be much more enjoyable.

Rain

As with the wind, you always have a choice to not ride if it's raining. There's no shame in ducking out of a gray, wet day. But if you are touring on a group ride or get caught in a cloudburst, you won't have much of a choice. The wet can quickly suck your energy because your body consumes so much more of it to keep itself warm when soaked. The best defense against rain is to watch the weather and grab rain gear before you head out if the forecast looks dicey.

Wet roads not only make it harder to hold your traction, they also make you take longer to slow down in an emergency and make it much more difficult to catch the attention of passing motor vehicles because of decreased visibility. Increase your chances of being seen by wearing bright clothing, extra reflective gear, and lights.

Snow and Ice

It's best to avoid riding in either of these conditions, but if you live in more northern climates and want to commute through the winter, you may not have a choice. Ice is inherently dangerous and not really rideable. If you want to venture out in the snow, your best bet is to invest in studded bicycle tires. After that, just put extra care into maintaining your bike. Winter conditions can wreak havoc on moving parts.

CHAPTER 23

Emergency Maneuvers: The Martial Arts of Cycling

LIKE MANY OF THE MARTIAL ARTS, THE REAL TRICK TO SURVIV-ing a fight with an unknown and unexpected opponent is to be on the defense. It takes less energy to react than to attack because you can use the power of that attack to your advantage. Although there's not much that's great about unexpected dangerous situations, getting out some cones and practicing these maneuvers until they're second nature will give you a great boost in your bike-handling skills. When that emergency comes up, you won't even think, you'll just avoid.

Emergency Stop

Emergency stops can manifest themselves in these common scenarios: the car that suddenly backs out of a driveway, the light that turns red, or the irresponsible driver who throws litter out of the window of his car. They are also easy to learn because they are mainly an exaggeration of your normal braking technique. After putting both your feet evenly on the pedals, grab a handful of both your brakes. This isn't the time for feathering: Go big or go down. Simultaneously shift your butt so far back that you're behind the saddle and thrust your arms forward. This will cause your torso to drop down over the top tube and lower your center of gravity, which will keep you glued to the road. Be bold as you force your bike forward and push your weight back. (See image on page 117 for an example.)

Road Kill Roundabout

The dreaded road kill—unfortunately, it will happen eventually. Whether it's the victim of wildlife, a big rock, or random garbage, there will be things in the road you want your tires to miss but you don't see until it's too late to ride around. You can still figure-eight the path of your wheels around them. Ride until you're a few inches short of the obstacle and then quickly steer left then right, then continue riding on past the debris. When you flick your handlebars, the bike will lean each direction and your tires will roll around it. This is a great

(*continued on page 138*)

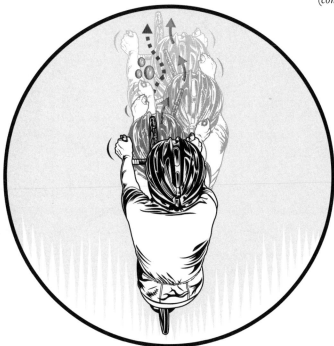

Tracking your front wheel quickly to the right and left of the obstacle will help make a figure eight with your wheels around it, so you miss it completely.

Giving Road Hazards the Runaround

SURFACE HAZARDS

Hazard: Debris like piles of broken glass; gravel after a winter storm; fallen tree branches; piles of leaves; nasty, sunken sewer grates; and potholes

Ride Around: These are best avoided with good scanning techniques so you can move out of their way ahead of time. If you can't avoid them, stand up on your pedals and relax your arms and legs. Don't hit the brakes, as momentum is more likely to help you cruise over them.

Hazard: Wet leaves or wet metal (steel plates, manhole covers)

Ride Around: Brake and slow down before rolling over them. When your tires make contact, don't pedal or brake at all. Coasting will glide you over, but any friction control (like accelerating or hitting the brakes) will cause your wheels to slide out.

Hazard: Railroad tracks

Ride Around: Always cross the tracks as close to 90 degrees as possible. By making your path perpendicular to the ruts, you're less likely to fall into them. Also, use the techniques for debris and wet metal if the tracks are raised or rutted.

VISUAL HAZARDS

Hazard: Obstruction of view like fences, bushes, buildings, and parked vehicles

Ride Around: Slow down and take extra caution until the line of sight is clear.

Hazard: Rain

Ride Around: Remember that you and the vehicles have decreased awareness and less traction—a really bad combo. Ride a little slower than normal, take longer to slow down, and make yourself as visible as possible with bright clothing or lights.

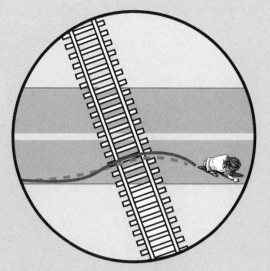

Always cross railroad tracks at a right angle.

Hazard: Dawn, dusk, and the sun

Ride Around: Remember that everything is harder to see at these times of day because of diffused light or, worse yet, the sun in the eyes of people driving around you. Use extra caution during these hours. Keep in mind, most people are either just waking up and heading to work or tired from a full day of punching the clock. Either way, ride as if drivers might be a little spacey.

COLLISION HAZARDS

Hazard: Dogs, kids, squirrels, and the cats that chase them

Ride Around: For any of the above, keep them in your peripheral vision in case they make a kamikaze run for it into the road. With dogs, be especially watchful of owners who use retractable leashes. They're instant clotheslines for unsuspecting cyclists.

Hazard: Other cyclists

Ride Around: If riding on a shared path or in a group ride event, you'll be cycling with people who may have no idea how to ride with others. Keeping this in mind, slow down and have a bell or call out a warning of "On your left!" before overtaking them.

Hazard: Motor vehicles

Ride Around: Keep an eye out for cars exiting or entering driveways or other turns. If it looks like a car is slowing but isn't signaling, assume it is going to turn anyway and wait to see what it does before proceeding. The bottom line: It's always better to be safe than sorry.

one to practice with a rag or something you can easily roll over. You'll be surprised at how quickly you can make this move—and how easy it is to stay upright.

Hop Like a Rabbit

The bunny hop is a classic move that not only helps you get over cracks in pavement and pot-holes, but also looks cool while you're doing it and makes you feel like a kid again, too. Crouch down like a tiger, elbows out, knees bent, feet even, butt back and off the saddle. Get as close as you can to the pothole, and then, as if you're leapfrogging with your bike, spring up with your body while pushing your bars slightly for-ward. Without enough momentum, your hop won't be long enough to clear both wheels, so hold some speed to make this happen. As you land, keep your joints bent and your booty off the saddle to absorb the landing.

Dog Daze

Dogs are man's best friend and less commonly known as a cyclist's nightmare. If you're riding on a shared bike path, slow down and warn owners early that you're coming up on them with a call of "On your left!"—especially if they have a retractable leash that can clothesline you. This will give them time to get their canine under control so you can ride safely by.

Unfortunately, out in the countryside, you'll have less luck with leash laws or having an owner actually being present. If a loose canine comes tearing after you barking its head off, you have a host of options to get away safely. Most of the time, dogs are either playing or trying to protect their territory. Either way, they're not much of a threat if you ignore them and carry on—without speeding up. Dogs love nothing better than a game of chase, so if you accelerate, they may think it's an invitation to play.

If they do get too close, slow down, stay calm, use your deepest, sternest "bad dog" voice, and tell them firmly to go home. Don't scream in panic. Don't try to kick or hit them. Dogs react to your temperament, so fearful reactions or timid voices tell them they need to be fearful themselves and will consequently incite further barking and raise their excite-ment level.

If they are still on your wheel, spray them with your water bottle. This usually does the trick, but if your regular route is a plague of pooches, an air horn or a non-toxic dog deter-rent like Spray Shield are great options. These work as well as pepper sprays, but won't affect you if the wind happens to be blowing the wrong way.

Sometimes just stopping, putting the bike between you and the dog, and waiting for the owner is the best tactic.

If You're Going Down ...

Sometimes there's no avoiding an accident. If you are certain you're going down, don't stick your arm out to try to break your fall—that's the shortest route to broken bones. Instead, hold on to the handlebar, tuck your head and shoulder, and try to land on large muscle masses such as your bottom, hip, or shoulder. Angling your body toward the ground, use the flow of the energy to dissipate the impact and try your best to roll out of the fall. Of course, if your helmet has impact—no matter how hard—it's going into retirement. Don a fresh one for your next ride. Bonus: You'll feel safer and more confident for your post-wreck return to the road.

CHAPTER 24

Expecting the Unexpected: What to Do in Case of an Accident

THE ONE BEAUTIFUL THING ABOUT FALLING IS THAT YOUR body will immediately respond by flooding your system with a wonderful, magical drug called adrenaline. It will make you feel a huge surge of energy and will take away a good amount of any pain you have. Its job is to temporarily make you feel like everything is fine and dandy. The more extensive the injury, the more powerful the surge your body will send. Although fantastic, you just have to keep in mind that most likely, everything is not okay and you won't know for sure until the adrenaline wears off and you see a doctor. As with any drug, you don't want to be riding—or making decisions—while intoxicated.

If You Fall

DON'T GET RIGHT UP. Give yourself a moment on the ground to check yourself over. Broken bones often don't hurt more than bruises or sprains.

DON'T EXPECT TO RIDE HOME. On your way to work for that big meeting? Your husband's birthday party is tonight? Time to make alternate plans. Right now you may need a ride home or a trip to urgent care to get checked over.

KEEP WARM. If it's cold out, put on a jacket if you don't already have one. Adrenaline and shock go hand and hand, so you'll lose your body warmth quickly if it's cold.

DRINK WATER. This will help your body equalize the adrenaline surge. It also gives you something to do and burns the excess energy.

ACCEPT HELP. No matter what the cause, it's embarrassing and a little humiliating to find yourself on the ground. But don't let your ego (and adrenaline) convince you that you're a hero and can take care of yourself. If other people offer to check your bike or give you a lift, take them up on it. Usually others are a better judge of how hurt you are—often because you can't see how bad your scrapes and bruises are.

IF YOU HIT YOUR HEAD, DO NOT KEEP RIDING. Head injuries are serious business. You are as likely to have a concussion from a secondary bump as you are from a direct impact—and either way your helmet has been compromised. Get a lift.

If You Are Hit by a Vehicle

FOLLOW THE ABOVE GUIDELINES AND . . .

STAY CALM. That adrenaline? It can also make you get very angry or upset with the driver—especially if he or she caused the crash. Sometimes disorientation will also cause you to apologize profusely—even if it wasn't your fault. Don't apologize or accuse, concentrate on taking care of yourself and your bicycle.

CALL THE POLICE. In some states or cities they may not come out to the scene, in others they'll be there in a flash. Either way, plan on filing your own accident report at the DMV within 36 hours.

GET THE DRIVER'S INFO. This means exchange names, driver's license numbers, registration, insurance, and any other info you would get if two motor vehicles were involved.

SAVE YOUR FILES. If you're carrying a computer or phone that tracks your route with GPS, save the file as evidence in case of future disputes.

GET INFO FROM WITNESSES. On TV, the cops would do this for you, but in reality it's your job to secure eyewitnesses. If someone saw the incident, get his or her name and contact info.

IF THE DRIVER FLEES . . . try to get the vehicle make, model, license plate number, and a description of the driver. Try to find eyewitnesses. In all states it's a federal crime to leave the site of an accident you were involved in, and moves the severity up to "hit-and-run" status. Still call the police.

PART VII

WELL, HOW DO YOU DO? ROAD ETIQUETTE

Don't be that person. You know, the one no one likes to ride with because you just don't get how to ride with other people? That one. Like any good relationship, there's both an art and a science to riding with other cyclists. It's one part predictability, one part courtesy, one part humility, and one part working for the group. It doesn't matter if you're riding with your best friend, touring with your significant other, or racing with your team. Even if you're riding solo, these social rules help keep your fellow cyclists (present or not) safe by setting a good example for them and for drivers.

CHAPTER 25

Rules of the Road

YOUR RULES OF THE ROAD WILL VARY STATE BY STATE, SO TO find out yours, go to your local DMV or ask your statewide bike advocacy group. Most provide information on their websites or can send you a pamphlet. No matter where you ride though, there are some general road rules that are universal.

Be Predictable

Nobody feels safe around the car that's swerving all over the lane, not using signals, acting all crazy by suddenly stopping or accelerating in odd places with no warning. Ride as you would drive—as if you were trying to pass a driver's license test.

Follow the Laws

In most states, bikes are treated like vehicles (and ticketed accordingly). When riding in the road, always signal, make complete stops at signs, and wait for red lights and your turn to maneuver.

Ride to the Right

Always ride with the flow of traffic—to the right. However, if there is no shoulder and you're riding on a two-way street, it's always safer to stay in the imprint of the right car wheel well in the road. This will keep you on the right but far enough left to be more visible and avoid opening doors from parked cars. It also forces cars behind you to move into the oncoming lane to pass you, making them slow down and give you more room—a win/win situation.

If you're transitioning for a left turn, you'll want to move from the right to the middle of the lane or merge into the left turn lane if available. Make sure to check over your left shoulder for oncoming traffic and signal left before moving over to your new position in the road.

Share the Road

Whether it's with cars, pedestrians, or your fellow cyclists, be courteous. Keep in mind that being on the road is a privilege, not a right.

Be a Defensive Rider

When it comes down to it, in a conflict on the road, most motor vehicles around you will win. You may have the law of the land on your side, but the laws of physics are on theirs. Keep an eye out for dangerous, unpredictable riders; drivers; and road hazards.

Wear a Helmet

Although it isn't mandatory in most states for adults to wear helmets, it's always a smart idea that can save your life. This is a no-brainer.

Avoid Riding on Sidewalks

Terrible sight lines and people entering and exiting doorways and driveways mean riding on sidewalks is an accident waiting to happen. If you find yourself forced onto the sidewalk, slow to a speed no faster than most people could jog—about 6 to 8 miles per hour—until you can get back on the road.

CHAPTER 26

Road Ragin'

WHEN BEHIND THE WHEEL OF A MOTOR VEHICLE, PEOPLE
sometimes turn into the worst versions of themselves. Perfectly reasonable, sweet
people—good neighbors, favorite aunts, your brother-in-law—are unfortunately not
immune to this phenomenon. Perhaps you've even experienced it yourself? A sudden,
unexpected overreaction to another driver's small slight is perceived as a huge, inten-
tional, and uncalled for assault on you, your car, your entire day, and your personal
happiness. Unreasonable? Yes. But as cyclists on the road, we're more vulnerable in
these kinds of confrontations. Sometimes we can even incite them with our own less-
than-courteous behavior while on the road.

The best policy is that if an accident was avoided, just practice patience and let it
go. You may be tempted to exchange words with the driver, which is okay as long as
they seem willing to connect and you're approaching them calmly, with respect and
consideration (even if you don't think they deserve it), to ask them to be more careful
or courteous. Some great conversations have started this way—as long as they are
exactly that. Approaching anyone—a vehicle, pedestrian, or other cyclist—in anger,
frustration, or fear will *never* end well. Even if you are calm, cool, collected, and open,
it can still sometimes end badly. Remember that drivers with road rage are at the
present moment the worst versions of themselves, so think twice about approaching
them at all.

If a driver is using his vehicle to threaten you, injure you, force you off the road, or is throwing objects at you (yes, these all rarely but occasionally happen), call 911 and report him as driving drunk and/or menacing. Most police want these kinds of drivers off the street as much as you do, and it's possible that kind of erratic or violent driving is because the driver is intoxicated or otherwise in a state where he shouldn't be behind the wheel. By reporting the make, model, and hopefully license plate of these drivers, you're doing your part to make the road safer for everyone.

CHAPTER 27

When Nature Calls

HOPEFULLY AT THIS MOMENT YOU'RE NEAR A GAS STATION OR restaurant. But often the best roads to ride are in the middle of nowhere, so if you have to go, do so discreetly. You wouldn't want to find people relieving themselves on your lawn, so do others the same courtesy. Find a place sheltered from the road and away from homes and places of business. There's going to have to be some level of undress—especially for the ladies—so try to be out of any line of sight. If necessary, your fellow riders can screen the road for you and serve as lookouts for cars. Although this is a natural bodily function, there are always those who are easily offended. In many states, the punishment by law for public urination can be anywhere from a ticket to an arrest, so keeping a low profile is the safest—and most polite—option.

CHAPTER 28

Pleasantville: The Nod, the Finger, the Wave, the Smile

YOU'RE RIDING ALONG AND YOU SPY AN ONCOMING CYCLIST. IT doesn't matter if you don't know him, or that he's in full pro kit, or his bike is an upright clunker, or it's just a kid riding to her neighbor's house. The friendly thing to do is say hello. The road is an unruly place sometimes, so add a little brightness to your day and hers by acknowledging her existence and the shared joy of being on a bike at the same time. A long held cycling adage is that it's always better to have a crummy day on the bike than no day on the bike at all, so keep this in mind when you see others on two wheels.

If you're in a pain cave and can barely make out that a bicyclist is in your field of vision, a gentle nod and smile will do. Hands need to be on the bars for safety? Just

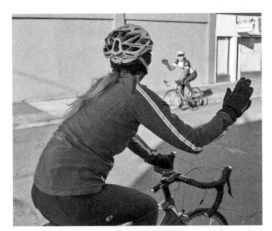

A simple hello and acknowledgment of others on the road can go a long way.

lift your index finger and flash those pearly whites. Riding along on the flats? Go ahead and give a nice friendly wave and a grin. It helps not only to connect but is always a good reminder that we should never take cycling (or ourselves) too seriously. After all, at the end of the day we're really just big kids on bikes.

It may not come as a surprise that there is occasionally animosity between people behind the wheel of a car and those on two wheels. A friendly wave or smile is also a good technique to use when vehicles are courteous enough to pass you with extra caution or wave you through a stop sign. If a driver is being less than kind to you as a cyclist, or just has the idea that anyone on a bicycle is a menace to society and should be riding on the sidewalk, use the same techniques. Killing them with kindness is a powerful tool and no matter how you feel about being treated less than respectfully, you can catch more flies with honey than vinegar. Who knows? You might just even change the mind of one of those drivers so that they give the next cyclist a little more leeway.

Remember, we're all out here sharing the road—it's just that some of us are lucky enough to be having fun doing it.

CHAPTER 29

The Hive Mentality: How to Ride (and Survive) in a Group

GROUP RIDING BASICALLY ENCOMPASSES ANYTIME YOU'RE NOT riding solo, and it comes with its own set of challenges: Now you're not only riding for yourself, but also for the good of the entire group. However, not all groups are the same. A 3-day bicycle tour with your best friends is going to roll differently from a ride with a seasoned racing team, and an organized fun-ride with 200 strangers is going to ride another way altogether. Still, there are many techniques that will apply to any group riding situation.

Clear communication and expectations are essential to group harmony. Don't assume everyone is on the same page. If you show up for a ride with your buddies with tired legs and only want to ride flat for 30 miles, it's important to know that the woman who called the ride together is looking to lead an all-day epic. Full disclosure from the ride organizers (even if that's just you and a friend) goes a long way. Sometimes that may mean you pedal a little slower or faster than you're comfortable with for the greater good of keeping the group together and the ride moving forward. If you're not on board with the plan for the day, you may want to go for a spin on your own.

Although you're keeping in mind the welfare of the group, don't slack off into being a lemming that just follows along without thinking. It's important to take care of yourself and think as an individual, as well as speak up for what you need—like a break or to slow down a bit. If the group or leader is attempting something scary or potentially hazardous, you don't have to follow. At the end of the day, no matter who's in front of you, you're ultimately responsible for your own well-being.

Riding in a group or pack can also help you learn valuable individual riding skills that you may not be able to otherwise master. There's a big difference between reading about how to climb and seeing someone dance on the pedals up a hill. This is the ultimate "monkey see, monkey do." Watching others execute proper technique helps our brains and muscles understand what good form looks like.

Unofficial Group Rides with Friends, Clubs, or Teams

Unofficial group rides come in many flavors, from weekly club rides to team training rides to Saturday spins with a few close friends. They are usually designated into one of two groups: drop or no-drop. Being "dropped" is the somewhat unpleasant term for getting left behind to fend for yourself and find your way home. A "no-drop ride" implies that the group will wait for you if you get a flat or fall off the back of the group.

Sometimes a team or club will differentiate what kind of ride it is when advertising them, but if not, it's a really good idea to ask. If you're uncomfortable with finding the route or catching up from a mechanical problem, don't head out on a no-drop ride unless you can find a buddy that's willing to stick with you.

Newer riders tend to either ride alone or stick to no-drop rides. Rides where everyone stays together tend to be more recreational and less aggressive than rides where you can be left to fend for yourself. That being said, joining a regular ride that hammers along without stopping can be a great challenge and can help you build speed and stamina. Because these rides that don't wait for stragglers tend to be a bit more competitive, they will push you harder and faster and be a great motivator for getting in

(continued on page 156)

Group Riding Decoder Ring

AFTER DECIDING HOW FAR AND FAST the group will be going, it's very important to keep those phone lines open while you're out on the ride. When you're riding close together, one person hitting a rock or pothole can have a dangerous cascade effect on the rest of the riders, who only have a limited view of the road. If you're the leader or there are riders behind you in a pack, it's considered not only polite but also responsible to let them know what lies ahead. The shout-out is nice, but keep in mind the other riders may not be able to hear you over traffic or wind noise. Always use sign language and fall back on using a verbal warning only if there's not enough time (or it's not safe) for you to signal.

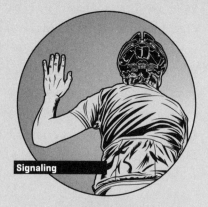

Signaling

SIGNALING

SIGNAL WHEN YOU'RE COMING UP for a turn or changing lanes.

   The Shout-Out: "Right," "Left," or "Turning"

   Sign Language: Pointing right or left with a straight arm parallel to the ground. You can also use the driver's education version of hand signals—point left with a straight left arm, or stick your left upper arm straight out and lift your lower arm 90 degrees so your hand sticks straight up and your arm looks like a right angle.

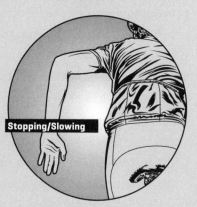

Stopping/Slowing

STOPPING OR SLOWING

THIS CAN HELP AVOID A NASTY multi-bike pileup.

   The Shout-Out: "Slowing" or "Stopping"

   Sign Language: Put your left upper arm straight out and drop your lower arm from the elbow to make a right angle that faces down. Also, with either arm angled straight down toward the ground and the palm of your hand facing behind you, swing your arm gently backward a few times.

POTHOLES, GRAVEL, ROCKS, AND FOREIGN OBJECTS

ANYTHING YOU WANT TO AVOID riding over falls into this category.

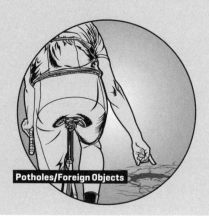

Potholes/Foreign Objects

The Shout-Out: Call out whatever the obstacle is.

Sign Language: This is probably where you see the most variety of signs. All of them generally point to the object. If it's scattered and spread out—like gravel or glass—the riders will often spread their palm flat to the ground and shake it back and forth.

NARROWING ROADS, PARKED CARS, PASSING PEDESTRIANS

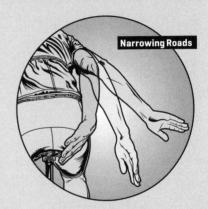

ANYTIME YOUR PATH OF TRAVEL IS significantly altered— for example, by the shoulder disappearing or a car being parked in it—you'll use this signal.

The Shout-Out: "Narrowing" (rarely used)

Sign Language: With a straight arm pointed behind you, swipe your hand toward the direction riders need to move.

PASSING

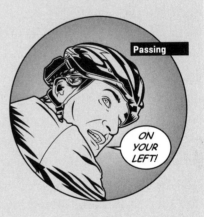

SOMETIMES YOU'LL WANT TO OVERTAKE cyclists or pedestrians from behind. Because they can't see what you're doing, it's important to warn them you're passing before you line up with the back of their wheel since they likely won't be expecting it. Always pass on the left.

The Shout-Out: "On your left!" is better than "Passing!" but the best is a ring of a bell.

CARS FROM BEHIND

THIS IS THE MOST IMPORTANT and consistently used warning to other riders, and it's the one time that the riders from behind hold the responsibility.

The Shout-Out: "Car back!"

Sign Language: None, since the riders being warned can't see behind them.

better shape if you're cycling for fitness or with aspirations of racing.

Organized Group Rides

In these events you'll pay an entry fee to pedal along with somewhere between 50 and 5,000 like-minded riders along a marked, predesignated route with support vehicles and rest stops provided by the organizers. Usually these one- to multi-day events are fundraisers or designed around a particular theme or location, and you have the added benefit of not having to worry about food or route-finding—the organizers take care of the details for you. Although everyone wants to have a great time, since you've likely never met most of the riders around you, everyone will have their own version of what that means. Some cyclists are out to challenge their past year's performance for a personal best time. Others might just be trying to get to the finish of their first long ride or have a fun day with friends or family. These different agendas can butt up against each other, but there are a few simple ways to keep the peace.

Hopefully the organizers have given you a map, cue sheets, and marked turns along the route. Now it's up to you to ride courteously and generously with all your new cycling compatriots. Use all your signals and communications. When passing, give plenty of loud warning before you pass, then plenty of room as you do ride by. A startled cyclist is an unpredictable cyclist—and prone to swerving. Yelling a warning when you're already right up next to them may do more harm than good. Never, ever pass on the right, even if the cyclist is in the middle of the road. By giving them plenty of warning, they should have time to move over. If it takes them a second, keep your patience and slow down until it's safe to pass—which shouldn't be a big deal if you're already that much faster than them. Anytime you make a pass, it's nice to give a thanks, a wave, or a quick "Have a great ride!" before carrying on.

If you're the one being passed, move over as soon as it's safe. Don't hold a grudge or take it personally that someone is faster than you and make it more difficult to pass than need be. If you're already over toward the right side of the road, continue to hold your line and don't make any sudden moves to the right or left that could throw off other riders around you.

Touring

If you think you want to bike tour with someone, make sure that you not only have ridden with them before but that you are also on the same page as far as expectations for speed, stops, and mileage. Take the story of Ellee Thalheimer, author of the cycle touring guide *Cycling Sojourner* and the *Lonely Planet Guide to Italy*, and her then fiancé (now husband), Joe Partridge. Joe was a long-distance endurance racer without much touring experience, and Ellee loved nothing more than eating, drinking, and breathing adventure on two wheels—but at a steady pace with plenty of stops. Two strong, experienced cyclists hitting the road together—a perfect match. Before they set out on their first tour, it was decided that they'd ride close together for the most part, except on climbs (where Joe was much stronger), when they would regroup on the top.

It quickly became clear by the end of the first day that while Ellee was content to stop, take photos, eat a leisurely lunch, and take her time pedaling through their predetermined mileage, Joe was in race mode and getting frustrated with what he felt was puttering along. Joe's lunch was a quickly woofed-down energy bar. Ellee pulled out an avocado, some bread, hummus, nuts, and veggies. Joe, not only exasperated, was also a little jealous.

After a big discussion at the campground that first night, it was decided that someday Ellee would enter an endurance race, but in the meantime, Joe was going to learn to take the world in a little more slowly. Their story has a happy ending. Joe learned that there can be a lot more to touring than bagging miles (including lots of off-the-beaten-path adventuring), and Ellee later found that she was a fantastic endurance racer when she was one of the few finishers of a 200-mile race on gravel roads in 110-degree heat.

The moral here is that if you're planning on touring with other people and want to stick together, you'll want to have very compatible riding paces and goals, or the faster person will have to slow down to the pace of the slowest person in the group. You can also decide to follow the same route and not actually ride together, but meet up at the end of the day—which some people find to be the way to go so that each rider can enjoy the day at his or her own pace.

Pack Riding and Pacelines

The main difference between riding as a group and working as a pack is the use of drafting, where you get very close to the rider ahead of you—optimally less than a foot behind them—and the aerodynamics of their body breaking the wind pulls you along. You can do this with just two cyclists, with 20, or with an entire race like in the Tour de France. It's a great tactic to make it through windy days or very long rides and very, very useful to new cyclists who may not be as strong as their fellow pack riders.

The most organized pack riding happens in pacelines, where riders conform to one or two (called a double) long lines. Cycling in a properly functioning paceline can be a huge thrill. It's the epitome of working together for a larger

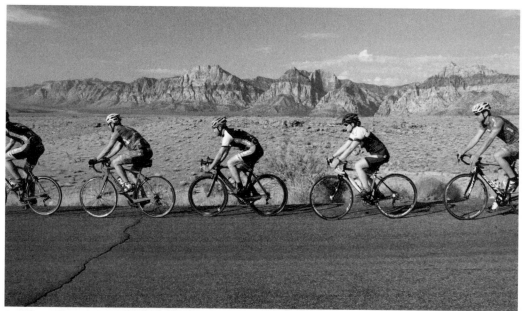

A well-organized paceline can be a beautiful, exciting, and fast time on the bike.

cause. The workload is shared as each rider takes his turn at the front—called a pull. This allows a peloton to sometimes ride 5 or more miles per hour faster than an individual could solo. It's pretty cool to be swept along—and keep up—with a group of riders and can make the miles spin by so much more smoothly.

Unfortunately, sometimes the paceline can be more effort than it's worth if the riders aren't playing nice with the rest of the group or, worse yet, don't know the rules well enough to participate. In these cases, the ride quickly deteriorates into both a figurative and literal drag. Following these basic rules and etiquette will get you far and have your group performing like a finely tuned machine.

Close and Predictable

After you've mastered the basic skills of shifting, braking, riding comfortably with one hand, and, most importantly, staying steady in a dead-straight line (even when grabbing your water bottle), you can work on pack riding. Start by working your way in closer to the rider ahead of you. Riding a foot from the wheel in front of you can be intimidating at first, so practice one-on-one with a friend starting at a bike length behind and whittle away at the gap a little bit at a time. You won't really feel the benefits of the draft until you're about a wheel's-length away—however, never get so close that your wheel comes even with or ahead of the wheel in front of you. This is the number one cause of crashes because it doesn't leave room for reaction time or for the forward rider to swerve around debris.

Heads Up

It's tempting to want to look at the rear of the rider ahead of you or, worse yet, stare at their wheels. It's also a very bad idea. Always keep your head up and your eyes trained as far ahead on the road as possible. This will not only help when there's a hazard in the road, but also gives you an early warning to the pack slowing or picking up speed. In your peripheral vision, mind the gap in front of you and the legs of the riders ahead. If you see them slow in pedaling or sit up to the top of their bars (which is a great way to slow without hitting the brakes), the pack speed is decreasing or you might be heading down a descent, while faster pedaling might signal that the pack is about to pick up some speed.

Smooth Like Butter

To keep the group formation together and riding gracefully, you'll need to pedal as smoothly as possible. Shifting regularly to maintain a higher cadence (faster pedal stroke) helps even out your acceleration and makes it easier to make micro-adjustments in the constantly changing speed within the pack. At a lower cadence, it's too easy to fall behind and then surge ahead, making the whole group spread out and bunch up like a rolling Slinky. Ulti-

mately, the goal is to ride as a cohesive machine and stick close together.

Brake with Caution

Braking can blow up a tight pack—and slamming on the brakes when another rider is drafting you can be disastrous. To respond to subtle decreases in speed when you're coming too close to the rider in front of you, soft-pedal lightly for a few strokes. Sitting up a little to catch more wind can be just as effective. If you do need to use your brakes, feather them gently while continuing to pedal lightly.

Find Your Place

The paceline's rhythm is for one rider to take a pull at the front until they feel fatigued (between a half-mile to a few miles), then peel off and drift back to the back, allowing the next rider in line to move up into the pulling position. This way, the load of keeping the pack moving steadily is shared and no one tires out too quickly. From front to back, each part of the pack has different stresses put on it, and there are positions to avoid when you're first learning how to ride well with others.

THE FRONT RIDER is doing the most work, pulling the rest of the group along and breaking the wind for them. This is the toughest and most important position to be in because it takes the most strength and attentiveness. It's the responsibility of the front rider to hold the pace as steady as possible and warn other riders of changes in direction or road hazards. When the front rider needs a break, he peels off—usually to the left—sits up, and coasts until he finds his position at the back of the line. Pulling at the front is usually left to the strongest and more seasoned riders who are most aware of their limits. Pulling for too long can leave the rider too fatigued to hold on to the pack after his turn at the front is over.

The lead rider also has to control the speed of the pack both up and down hills. It's tempting at the front to power into a descent, but any surge—even downhill—can string the group out. On the front, you want to coast on the descents and not attack on the climbs—otherwise the front of the group will have to soft-pedal and wait for the back. That being said, there are always long climbs that will splinter the group. It's the responsibility of the whole pack to regroup at the top and make sure no one is left too far back.

THE SECOND RIDER IS AS IMPORTANT AS THE FIRST. It's essential for the pack to maintain as close to the same pace as possible. When the first rider peels off, the next rider back will need to pick up his effort because he's just lost his wind block. The trick is to do this without actually picking up any speed, so someone in the middle of the pack wouldn't even notice the change in leadership. The front rider upping the pace—either from ego or a rider overestimating how hard to pull to keep the pack rolling—is a common mistake that results in blowing the line apart. Either way, the goal is to stay together, and sudden accelerations—even of just 1 or 2 miles per hour—can pop riders off the back. Keep an eye on the group's speed by checking in with your computer regularly, and when it's your turn to pull, maintain that pace.

You may not be able to take a pull when the overall speed of the group is near your limit, but that doesn't mean you can't ride in a paceline. If you're too tired (or not yet strong enough) to take your turn, immediately pull off after the first rider has drifted back and is clear from your rear wheel. Stronger riders will gladly carry the group.

Don't try to be a hero. Letting guilt or ego keep you from skipping your turn to pull is a rookie mistake. Everyone knows what it's like to be the novice or slower person in the group. If you don't have the stamina that day to take the lead position, you'll just be slowing the pack's average speed down or risking popping yourself off the back by killing yourself during the pull—making the whole group wait for you. Wait for a day your legs feel fresh and strong before taking the lead. The most valiant team rider works for the greater good.

PULLING UP THE REAR might seem like a good, safe place for a new or slow rider to hide out, but sitting at the back of the paceline is actually pretty difficult—especially if there are more than five or six riders in the group.

Despite the lead rider's best efforts, a paceline is like a game of telephone: the tail-end rider will be the last to hear the news if the pack is slowing down or speeding up. The larger the pack, the bigger the gaps between riders, leaving the caboose of the train having to make sudden, high-effort adjustments to keep up or slow down. If you're a little slower than most of the group, the place to be is the middle of the pack.

MID-PACK IN A PACELINE IS THE SWEET SPOT. Here you can experience the cruise control and exhilaration the group effort brings and feel a little bionic—your superpowers fully realized. Your main job here is to stay on the wheel in front of you. The mid-pack positions are where riders rest and recover the most, taking time to freshen up for their next pull.

If you know you're in a group that's a bit faster than you and you're unlikely to ever be able to take a turn pulling, hanging out mid-pack is the place to be. If you rotate up toward the front, call out "Gap!" or just move over a little and wave a stronger rider behind you ahead to maintain your position. It's always okay to be the weak link. Every rider has been there at some point—and even experienced riders are smart to challenge themselves by heading out with a group that's faster. Being the "slow one" is made graceful by having humility to admit it and working as hard as you can to ensure the group stays as intact as possible.

PART VIII

NUTRITION: THE CARE AND FEEDING OF YOUR CYCLIST

On the bike, you'll be burning about 500 calories for each hour of pedaling, averaging around 12 miles per hour. "That's great!" you might think. "A quarter of the calories for my day—I can practically eat whatever I want!" Cue: cyclist pedaling straight for the doughnut shop.

It's easy to fall into the habit of throwing down a few extra cookies or beers at the end of the day as a reward for all the hard work you did on the bike. Unfortunately, sweets and alcohol aren't always the best fuel—or strength builders.

In taking a look at the ultimate foods for cyclists both on and off the bike, you can build a solid foundation to make your rides easier, find recipes for real foods that can make your riding miles fly by, and decide when it's time for that celebratory post-ride brew or something a little more fulfilling.

To give you the best nutrition and hydration advice, we've partnered up with Dr. Stacy T. Sims, an innovative exercise physiologist and nutrition scientist of thermoregulation, hydration, and performance nutrition, to give her expert advice on your nutrition needs. She's also the founder of OSMO nutrition products, which she developed to help solve the problems of gastrointestinal distress and hydration of athletes—including the Cannondale Pro Cycling Team.

Dr. Sims has spent her career researching and developing nutrition and hydration programs that have helped everyone from beginners to title-winning professional cyclists. Although most common-knowledge nutrition advice is based on studies of "professional male athletes ages 25 to 35," her groundbreaking research is some of the first to address what works best for women and active people outside of the old-school standard of narrowly defined boundaries.

CHAPTER 30

Getting Your Essentials

IT'S NOT THE NUMBER OF CALORIES CONSUMED, BUT HOW YOU consume them. Counting calories is an outdated form of knowing if you're eating too little or too much, and not very effective for your best cycling performance. Instead, start thinking of food in terms of what it can do for your body. On the bike, it gives you energy; off the bike, it helps your muscles and nervous system repair and rebuild for the next ride.

Some foods work better for fuel, others are great at helping you restore. Most importantly, as with bicycles, you want to grab the right component for the job at hand. It's less of a matter of "this is bad" or "this is good" than it is "this is a better fuel for storage, this is a better fuel for repair, and this is a better fuel for the next twenty miles." One of the best things about road cycling is that you can eat almost anything; it's just a matter of when, where, what, and how much.

Carbohydrates

Carbohydrates are where the magic is hidden—your main source for energy to burn for a body on the go. When you consume them, they are processed into glucose—a sugar that your blood carries to the muscles so that their cells can convert it into energy. Eat more than you're currently able to burn and your body will turn that glucose into long-term storage: fat.

Cyclists need carbs to get them through rides. This is the gas in your proverbial tank. However, not all carbs are built alike.

There are those that are complex. Some, like potatoes, bread, rice, and pasta, are what we often define as starches and are what usually come to mind when you hear the word "carbohydrate." When you think of a starch, it's usually a faster-burning fuel. Whole grains—oats, quinoa, brown rice—are also complex, but have more fiber and protein that release a slower, more even burn of energy.

There are also simple carbs like honey and sugar. What we typically think of as "sweets" are quickly converted to glucose because they are already essentially another type of sugar—which is also why they're easier to pack on the pounds with. Simple carbs also tend to have the least nutritional value. They are your body's straight source of octane, great for surges of energy, when you need to put the pedal to the metal.

Then there are foods that we don't typically identify as being carbs, because we don't see them next to the bread and pasta on the food pyramid. This includes milk (a simple carb), whole fruits (not juice or fruit sugars), vegeta-

Carbohydrates that Rock Your World

THESE ARE THE FOODS WITH THE MOST carbs and the best overall nutrition value. You may notice a theme—the foods with the most fiber are your best carbohydrate picks.

- ➤ Bananas
- ➤ Green vegetables
- ➤ Root vegetables
- ➤ Brown rice
- ➤ Quinoa
- ➤ Whole-grain bread and pasta
- ➤ Corn
- ➤ Pumpkin
- ➤ Legumes (beans, peas, lentils)
- ➤ Oatmeal
- ➤ Melon
- ➤ Apple
- ➤ Mango
- ➤ Berries

bles, and legumes like beans or peas (complex carbs). Fruits, veggies, and beans are great because they're full of energy as well as fiber, protein, vitamins, and minerals. Looking over the list above, it's clear to see that getting enough carbohydrates in your diet will usually never be a problem.

As a cyclist, you need every type of carbohydrate—but the key is to know what type and when to consume for the best energy source. Typically, slow-burning complex carbs are best at the dinner table. Starchy complex carbs (white rice, bread, or potatoes) are good on the bike as a medium-burning fuel to keep you running strong. If you're on an epic journey, or need to put out a hard effort for a short period of time, reach for the simple sugars your body can use quickly. Otherwise, choosing the carbs that are the least processed is usually the best.

Protein

If carbs are the fuel for your engine, protein is the lubricant: Without it, you'll burn out, no matter how much gas you have. Many people relate protein to bulking up—perhaps bodybuilders, football players, and power-based sports enthusiasts come to mind—but cyclists need it just as much, if not more so. And unlike carbs, your body can't store much protein for later use, so you need a consistent supply in your diet.

Although carbs are your primary source of energy, your body also utilizes a small but integral amount of protein to keep you pedaling strong—especially when your blood sugar is running low. Without it, your efforts will feel more arduous while your performance will decrease. More importantly, the hours you spend pedaling the bike—pushing up hills and chasing down your friends—do a number on your muscles. Your body needs protein to recover and rebuild so all that effort succeeds in making you stronger for your next ride. After riding, protein works to maintain and repair those hard-working muscle fibers and helps boost immunity. Without it, all your riding effort could be wasted.

Protein is also a primary brain food (so including it in your diet keeps you sharp) and helps suppress your appetite while revving up your metabolism because it takes more energy to digest. During endurance activities—like road cycling—it also lends itself to protecting vulnerable tissues and is critical for building up your immune system.

There are 20 different amino acids that can make up proteins, but foods that are protein-rich don't necessarily have all of them. Proteins are broken down into two groups: complete and incomplete. A complete protein contains all the essential amino acids your body needs for building, maintaining, and repairing muscles, and much more. Complete proteins include animal products—meat, dairy, and eggs—and soybeans.

Incomplete proteins are missing a few of the essential amino acids but make up for it by having higher levels of others. To get enough protein, you want to eat lots of other foods containing the complimentary amino acids. Incomplete proteins come from plant-based foods such as nuts, grains, and beans (although some, like the grain quinoa, are a complete protein on their own). It used to be thought that you needed to buddy up an incomplete protein with a complete one to make it whole. We now know that if you eat a wide enough variety of foods, it will still be enough—which is how vegetarian and vegan athletes are able to perform so well.

Fat Facts

The big "F." Fat is usually the bad guy—the villain of the story looming at our dinner table. Our culture cringes at the word when in fact we should embrace it. True, too much of some fats can foster disease and pack on pounds, ultimately decreasing our life expectancy. But a lot of fats are kinds that won't make us "fat," but instead are important sources of energy, full of essential types of acids that help our bodies stay healthy and protect us from disease. Not only that, but research has shown that athletes who include healthy fats as one-third of their daily diet are able to keep their stamina longer than those who eat a low-fat, higher-carb diet. They also tend to be leaner and have better immunity than those that follow a low-fat, high-carb diet.

What has fat ever done for you? For starters, it's an excellent source of fuel. Your muscles need more than just carbs and proteins, so adding fat to the mix gives you a third method of balancing your delicate glycogen stores and helps your body pedal at varying intensities so you can cycle longer without spiking and dropping your blood sugar levels. As your body becomes more fit from cycling, it also becomes a more efficient fat burner. Not only does this give you the ability to cycle longer and harder without crashing from low blood sugar, but it also keeps you from feeling as hungry.

Without fat, we can't absorb those cancer-fighting, immune-boosting antioxidants. You would also have a hard time producing or storing the estrogen and testosterone that help balance your nervous system and build nerve tissue if you were fat-free.

Here's what Dr. Stacy Sims has to say about our friendly fats: "Eating a diet containing a moderate amount of plant and nut sources of fat will not only improve your performance, but will also boost your immune system, help with muscle recovery, maintain even energy levels, and help you lean-up. The key to eating fat is that it increases satiation, thus you end up craving less sugar and other simple carbs and reducing cortisol (a.k.a. the belly-fat hormone) and overall body fat conservation. Word to the wise—choose 'natural fat' (avocados, nuts, seeds, olives) and avoid fat with sugar. The combination of fat with sugar increases your cravings for sugar, reducing the goodness of 'natural fat.'"

Like carbs and proteins, there are a variety of different kinds of fats out there, some of which are more helpful than others. Monounsaturated fats are sourced from nuts, avocados, and the oils of olives, canola, and nuts. Polyunsaturated fats are the rock stars of fatty acids, especially omega-3. These fatty acids have been shown to protect against some of the worst diseases plaguing Americans—like heart disease and diabetes—and might actually deter unhealthy fat storage. The best sources of fatty acids can be found in fish and flax seeds (which have become abundant on store shelves and in breakfast cereals).

Saturated fats have been recently redeemed after being singled out for years as bad guys. Found mostly in meats and dairy, they are what make everything from butter to cheese to lard so darned tasty—and the culprit behind the popular culinary trends in dishes like bone marrow, bacon, and foie gras. Although they aren't quite as evil as we were led to believe, you should still eat them in moderation since they can increase your risk of heart disease. The exception to this is coconut oil, which is plant-derived; scientists have discovered it acts more like an unsaturated fat in your body.

Finally, the lowlife of the family, trans fats. These kinds of fats should be avoided at all costs. Sound a little alarmist? Trans fats have been found to be the leading cause of artery hardening and clogs, and promote weight gain—even if you're not actually eating any extra calories. These are the cause of the dreaded inner tube of belly fat that increases your risk for heart disease and diabetes. Purely man-made and the poster child for overprocessing, they're created when you take a natural oil and hydrogen gas and solidify them together. If your ingredients include "hydrogenated oil," you're eating something that's so alien to your body that your digestive system freaks out and sends them straight to your bloodstream. Not good. If you do eat processed foods (and who doesn't, here or there?), make sure you read the labels. They're most often found in margarines, cookies, snack cakes, chips, crackers, and all that stuff that has been dialed in for deliciousness without a thought to our well-being.

Vitamins and Minerals

Although carbs, proteins, and fats keep your engine running, building up and maintaining your whole body as a fine-tuned machine takes a little more. Although taking a multivitamin can sometimes be helpful, these only account for a small segment of the nutrients your body needs. The beauty of whole foods (fruits, vegetables, legumes, whole grains, and other unprocessed foods) is that they go beyond supplying the basic nutrients that can be packaged into a pill.

One example is carotenoids, the most famous of which is beta-carotene. There are more than 500 different carotenoids that have been discovered, and scientists are always finding more. Inside the plant, these colorful compounds that give veggies their red, orange, and yellow colors help to photosynthesize light. In our bodies, they work together to create immune-boosting and disease- and inflammation-fighting combinations.

One surefire way of making sure you have enough is to keep your diet colorful. Red foods—cherries, tomatoes, and watermelon—can protect your skin from the sun's UV rays. Blue foods—beets, berries, red onion, and cabbage—can have an anti-inflammatory effect, promote circulation, and are chock-full of muscle-repairing antioxidants. Green foods—kale, broccoli, and spinach—can supercharge your body to help your blood carry more oxygen to your muscles, which keeps them from fatiguing and helps them bounce back

A Cyclist's Top Nutrient Playlist

CYCLISTS AND OTHER ATHLETES USE MORE of some nutrients than others. Here are our recommendations for the nutrients you need to have in your daily rotation to keep you working and playing strong on and off the bike.

IRON
What it does: FORMS RED BLOOD CELLS that carry vital oxygen to your muscles. Basically, it can make you faster.
Where you get it: Fish; lean meat; nuts; legumes; leafy greens; dried fruits; cooking in cast iron
Take note: Although vitamin C enhances absorption of iron, calcium blocks it by almost 60 percent, so eat your dairy and other high-calcium foods separately from your iron. Yep, that means your cheeseburger may not be as "healthy" as you'd hoped.

B VITAMINS
What they do: HELP CONVERT CARBS AND PROTEINS into glucose (your body's energy source) and are essential for cell repair
Where you get them: Dark, leafy greens; fish; legumes; low-fat dairy; whole grains (some breads and cereals are fortified with them)
Take note: Cyclists use up their supply of B vitamins when they exercise a lot, so boost these particularly when you're training or riding hard.

CALCIUM
What it does: BUILDS AND MAINTAINS BONES AND TEETH, helps regulate blood pressure, maintains healthy nerve function to keep your muscle fibers firing smoothly
Where you get it: Dairy; dark, leafy greens; calcium-fortified soy, nut, or coconut milks
Take note: Because cycling is a non-weight-bearing activity, there's no load or impact to signal bones to create density. If you're riding a lot, you may need higher than the recommended daily average dose of calcium and cross-train with a weight-bearing exercise. Otherwise, you may be at risk for low bone density, which causes fractures and osteoporosis.

after a hard day of riding. No matter where they fall in the rainbow, at the end of the day the key to helping your body do the best job possible is consuming a wide variety of fruits and veggies that will give you the best chance at getting all the nutrients you need.

Fiber

Protein isn't the only thing that can make you feel full. Fiber, the indigestible part of plants, is one thing you want to have plenty of in your diet.

VITAMIN C

What it does: BOOSTS IMMUNITY; BUILDS COLLAGEN, a building block for tendons and arteries; helps remove cell-damaging free radicals
Where to find it: Citrus fruits; tomatoes; bananas
Take note: This is one vitamin that is easily boosted with a supplement, but getting it from a processed source decreases the benefits you'll get.

VITAMIN E

What it does: INCREASES STAMINA AND ENDURANCE
Where to find it: Seeds; nuts; wheat germ; avocado
Take note: Like vitamin C, its healthful effects may be decreased significantly when you get it from a source other than whole foods.

POTASSIUM

What it does: HELPS MAINTAIN YOUR BLOOD'S acid/water balance and body's sodium levels
Where to find it: Potatoes; winter squash; avocado; yogurt; beans; leafy greens; dates; raisins; sports drinks
Take note: Though not usually from foods, it is possible to get too much potassium. It's helpful in sports drinks when you're losing most of yours to sweat, otherwise avoid extra potassium supplements and be careful of drinking too much coconut water, which has 20 percent of the recommended daily allowance of potassium per 6-ounce (yep, that's only half of most cans) serving.

MAGNESIUM

What it does: HELPS WITH ENERGY PRODUCTION and works with calcium for better smooth muscle contraction
Where to find it: Nuts; fish; beans; seeds; dark, leafy greens; dark chocolate
Take note: Magnesium can not only help you on the bike, but also helps your body balance and manage stress hormones so you stay chill all day long.

Insoluable fiber, found most often in fruits, vegetables, and whole grains, does not break down in water, but instead absorbs it, swelling in your digestive system and making you feel fuller, longer. Some examples include whole grains and bran, brown rice, vegetables (broccoli, green beans, corn), berries with seeds, fruits you can eat with skins on, and avocados and bananas. Since it's from the part of plants that give them their structure, you'll also get the benefits of eating foods that are high in nutrients. Because this fiber is indigestible, it slows down your system, allowing it to work more to get the good stuff into your bloodstream. You'll also need a lot more water to help your body with this process because insoluble fiber absorbs a lot of water.

Also from plants, soluble fiber forms a gel in water. It can be found in oatmeal, barley, and beans. High soluble fiber foods are great before a ride because they keep your blood sugar levels more sustained and stable. Some great high-fiber pre-exercise snacks include oatmeal (and oatmeal breads, cookies, muffins), beans, and legumes. Try some lentil soup with a side of whole grain bread, refried beans on a corn tortilla, or hummus with rye crackers. However, they're not the best foods to choose for when you're on the bike. They won't deliver the energy you need quickly enough and they sometimes can cause gastrointestinal distress (a.k.a. burping and passing gas).

CHAPTER 31

Water, Water Everywhere . . .

WATER SURROUNDS US AND IS CONTAINED WITHIN US—OUR
bodies are made up of 60 percent water. Even more so than food, water is the true
source of life and strength. We'd keel over quicker from a lack of water than a lack of
food. Yet even though we can easily sweat out a pound an hour—and up to two on hot
days—hydration is often the one thing most cyclists neglect. Which is too bad since
dehydration slows you down. A lot.

Dehydration is fluid loss that happens as you sweat from exertion. It's not just a
state that you suddenly end up in, but a continuum that starts from your very first
pedal stroke (sometimes earlier) and builds with every minute in the saddle that you
don't drink. Bear in mind, too, that your sweat doesn't just contain water but also
other valuable minerals called electrolytes that help your muscles function. You can
find these in abundance in foods, but sports drinks can help replenish them as well.
However, do your research. Not all sports drinks are created equal, and some are so
low in electrolytes that you might as well be drinking water.

In a state of dehydration, your body's ability to regulate heat fades, increasing your
core temperature and putting you in danger of overheating. Heavier cyclists will have
this effect amplified. At the same time, your blood volume decreases (making it a

thicker, slower flow), which puts a larger load on your heart. Essentially, the longer and more you sweat, the harder your ride gets and the worse you start to feel. Hot or windy days will make it worse, but less-conditioned riders who are new to the sport feel it most acutely.

The best way to start your ride is to be fully hydrated, and you can't simply accomplish this by slamming a couple pints in the few hours before. Only 10 percent of the water in your body is in your blood. The rest is in your muscles, organs, and bones—which count on blood-flow for their water supply. It takes almost a full day for your body to balance and replenish low levels. The water has to get delivered from your digestive system to your blood and beyond, so hydration isn't just something you need to be thinking about while you exercise, but in the 24 hours before your ride as well.

When you drink on the bike, you are simply trying to keep ahead of impending dehydration. It's impossible to fully hydrate while exercising, so rehydrating off the bike becomes especially critical if you're on a multi-day ride—like a bike tour, heavy training period, or the first nice weekend of the spring—because you won't have as much time to fully rehydrate.

Luckily, there are many ways to get the recommended 1½ to 2 quarts a day that our bodies need. You don't have to stick strictly to water. Almost any form of fluid is good—from juices, teas, and coffee to soups and the milk in your bowl of cereal. Don't overlook water-charged foods like melon, tomatoes, oranges, pears, cucumber, or celery—they count, too.

Avoid soda, sweetened drinks like flavored waters, and alcohol. All of these just add on the empty calories, and in the case of alcohol, actually dehydrate you. Thinking about diet soda or other artificial sweeteners? Not so great, either. Since your body doesn't really digest the processed chemical sweeteners, they may just prime your taste buds to eat more calorie-laden sweet stuff later. Studies have shown that for every "diet" drink consumed per day, the risk for being overweight jumps 41 percent. When in doubt, best to stick with good old water.

The Electrolyte Hype

Think of your body as a supercomputer of cells, tissues, and fluids that are constantly connecting and communicating through electrical impulses. It needs to maintain a delicately balanced environment, friendly to conduction, and that's where electrolytes come in. They are the salty rock-stars that keep those ions firing so your computer doesn't crash. On a ride, you know you're getting close to the danger zone when you feel cramping, fatigue, nausea, and possibly a little irrational or emotional. In short, it's important to keep your levels steady if you want to be strong on the bike and have a pleasant ride.

On a day-to-day basis, the foods we eat should give us plenty to keep our processors thrumming. When we jump on the bike and start to sweat, we leach them out—especially potassium and sodium, two of the seven main electrolytes our body needs. To keep things in balance, sports nutritionists have designed drinks to help replenish what we lose during a workout.

Although they've always been easy to find in food, electrolytes have been marketed since the creation of sports drinks and have gained in popularity with the advent of bottled waters and "energy drinks." Many of these contain carbohydrates as well, but the latest studies have said that on the bike, you should get most of your carbs from food and save your drinks for hydrating and digesting what you've eaten. Studies have found that this is a better way for your digestive system to absorb the most electrolytes and carbs possible. You can find electrolytes in drinks and foods lining your convenience store shelves and in towering displays at your local bike shop.

A good rule of thumb is to use them if you're working out in excessive heat or for over an hour of moderate exercise on the bike. Any less effort or time than that and water will work just as well and keep you from taking in more carbs than you need.

Be wary of trying to use gels for food that are marketed as "replenishing electrolytes." Because they are so dense in carbs, it takes a lot of water within your body to digest them. Instead of replenishing, they leave you more dehydrated. For this reason, gels are notorious for causing the infamous "gut rot," whose symptoms include cramping, bloating, and copious amounts of gas. If you do use gels, you need to drink a huge amount of water along with them to keep yourself from dehydrating during digestion.

CHAPTER 32

Everyday Eating: Setting Up for Success

IF YOU WANT TO HAVE A STRONG, SUCCESSFUL RIDING EXPERI-ence, it has to start at home. Your body is a complex system that prefers to run on healthy, natural foods. If fast food and processed, packaged meals are a huge part of your diet, you'll likely struggle when it comes time to pedal. Your body simply can't get the balanced nutrients it needs because the calories are devoid of real energy.

Cycling gives all of us a great incentive for eating healthy: It's called the *power-to-weight* ratio. This scientific term basically means the less weight you carry, the easier it is to pedal—especially up hills. This doesn't mean you should be starving yourself to get thin in the hope that you'll be the first to the top of the climb. In fact, it's just the opposite. If you undereat and don't keep your body stocked with calories, you'll lose weight but you'll be sacrificing your power in the saddle as well. Lucky for you, cycling while eating a healthy, balanced diet will make you stronger and help to shed some pounds.

There are a million excuses why you don't eat better. When it comes down to pushing the pedals, making healthier choices will not only better fuel you on the bike but also help make you feel supercharged all day long. That maple bar may look like a delicious energy boost, but in reality, it's likely to drag you down because it's the wrong ratio of what you need and in a less digestible form. Don't be fooled. We need carbs, fats, and sugars, but we need certain types more than others, and in the right proportions.

Fueling Up for Your Ride

If your ride is less than an hour and a half at an easy to moderate pace, you don't have to pay too much special attention to how to prepare your body. Just eat what you would on any regular, healthy day before.

The longer and harder you ride, the more it helps your performance (and how good you'll feel on the bike) for your body's gas tank to be as topped off as possible. If you're planning on riding longer than an hour and a half, you need to take care starting with how you eat the entire day before. It takes anywhere from 12 to over 24 hours for your body to fully digest food and stock up stores of glycogen that you need as you pedal. That means what you eat the day before is as—or more—important than what you eat the meal before a big ride. By stocking up the day before, you're ready for your ride with a full tank. Because digestion is a fairly long process, you don't want to try this the morning of, or

you'll just end up with a lead gut and valuable energy you could be using for your legs being taken up by your digestive system trying to break down breakfast.

A lot of people hear the term "carbo loading" and think that it's fair game to slam down as much pasta as you can the night before a big ride. But loading up doesn't mean eating a larger dinner than you usually would. Instead, think of it as dedicating a higher percentage of your meal to the carbs—but eating the same amount overall. It works best if you up your carbs a bit for 3 to 4 days before a big ride. For example, switch from two eggs to one and an extra piece of toast in the morning. Instead of heaping on plate after plate of pasta, have a small trout fillet pan-fried in olive oil with larger servings of rice and veggies than you might normally have and a serving of roasted sweet potatoes on the side. You'll build up your glucose reserves *and* your vitamins and minerals while giving your body a little protein to keep you muscles rested and in balance.

The morning of your ride, again focus on a higher-carb breakfast. Even though you were resting, overnight your body dips slightly into your glycogen stores, so you want to top them off one more time before you head out for a big ride or race. The key here is whatever you eat, make it easy to digest. Avoid high-fat meats—like bacon or breakfast sausage—and get your protein from a source that's also carb-rich, like yogurt or oatmeal. Give yourself a good dose of carbs in the form of cereal, pancakes, potatoes, or toast. Adding in light protein, like eggs or milk, will keep you satisfied a little longer. Whatever you do, stick with foods you enjoy and eat enough—around 400 to 550 calories' worth. Some of us will get race–day or club–ride performance jitters and won't feel like eating. The absolute worst thing you can do before a big ride is not eat breakfast.

If it's a while after breakfast or your last meal before your ride, it's good to add in a little pre-ride snack like a banana or an energy bar. Even something as simple as a handful of almonds can make a big difference. If you feel hungry, eat. Going into a ride well fueled will make it easier to push the pedals, plain and simple. Not only that, but studies have found that our bod-ies are smart little computers: You burn more calories after you've eaten than if you start exercising after fasting.

Getting Fluid

Since much of the water in your body is ingested through your small and large intestines and then carried through your blood to your mus-cles, where it's absorbed, it takes a while to become completely hydrated. Like filling your fuel tank, hydration is something you should work on starting the day before your ride because you can only absorb so much water in a short period of time.

Try to drink around 1½ to 2 liters the day before. When you wake up, start first thing

Dr. Sims's Rise-and-Shine Breakfasts

WANT TO BE AT YOUR BEST ON a big ride day? Try these recipes by Dr. Sims, who makes a living helping athletes eat and drink right to perform their best.

Her favorite pre-big ride meal:

BIRCHER MUESLI: Soak quinoa flakes and oatmeal overnight in almond milk with raisins. (Note: Quinoa flakes are the grain that has been rolled through a press. If you can't find them, substi-tute oatmeal or spelt flakes.) In the morning, dish up a bowl of the bircher muesli and top with fresh blueberries and raspberries, nonfat Greek yogurt, a sprinkle of walnuts, and a drizzle of honey. Have espresso on the side with a dash of cinnamon.

Second-best meal:

4-oz nonfat Greek yogurt, 1 Tbsp almond butter, 2 Tbsp avocado, 4 crushed summer-ripe straw-berries. Blend all together well. Spread over 2 slices of low-sugar, mixed-sprouted-grain toast.

with 0.18 to 0.2 ounces of water per pound of your body weight. Drink that same amount at least four more times throughout the day, concentrating on fluids like water, tea, coffee, or a little juice. Avoid sugary drinks like sodas or flavored coffees. Remember—you can drink a little less if you hydrate by eating water-heavy foods like fruits, veggies, or smoothies.

The day of your ride or race, start the day with a tall glass of water. Overall, make sure you get another 0.18 to 0.2 ounces of water per pound of your body weight before you hit the road—but this time add a dash of salt. "In the body, where water goes there is sodium; to improve the absorption of water, you need a bit of sodium," advises Dr. Sims. The sodium will also prevent you from having to hit the bathroom 10 times before the start of the ride because the water will stay in your body, where you need it most. Though it's important to hydrate on the bike as well, you'll be sunk if you start out in a deficit. It's simply impossible to catch up if you start behind, and being dehydrated is the quickest way to feel like crud on the bike—and the slowest to be able to bounce back from.

CHAPTER 33

On the Bike: Avoiding the Bonk

OH. THE DREADED BONK. IF YOU'VE NEVER HEARD THE TERM, it's usually uttered by cyclists under their breath when their rides go south. Most don't like to talk about it too loudly—as if not saying the word will avoid its onset. It is the nemesis of a good, fun ride.

Sound dramatic? Bonking is what happens when your body's levels of fuel or water (or both) gets too low. What does it feel like? Well, it not only affects your performance—though it can suddenly feel like you're pedaling through cement while someone has a rope attached to you pulling you backward. Your body will sag, and you'll feel like you can't force your legs to move. Worse yet, since your brain also runs on glycogen and needs to be hydrated to process things, you can feel confused, fuzzy-headed, angry, and desperate. Crying, swearing, or lock-jawed silence from your normally chatty friend is not unusual or an exaggeration of symptoms experienced while bonking.

The funny thing about it is that it's easily avoidable. Dr. Stacy Sims breaks it down for us. "There are two types of 'bonks.' One is the dead-leg fatigue that most people perceive as low calories; but really it is dehydration. This is the bonk you do not want to experience, as it takes hours to come back from dehydration. The second type is a true low blood sugar bonk. This is the light-headedness, tunnel-vision type of bonk that can be corrected easily with a bit of food and takes about 10 minutes to come right."

It really doesn't take much: Start hydrated and fueled, then eat and drink on the bike. Problem solved. But no matter how many times it's said, cyclists often have a strange compulsion to be the hero. If you didn't know, heroes don't eat, drink, or stop—ever. They have the mentality that if you need sustenance, well, you must be some kind of a wimp. It's the unspoken code of amateur cyclists. This is why bonking is so very, very common among us mere mortals aspiring to be heroes.

Of course, all the pros—those real heroes—know (and every book you read on nutrition, including this one, will tell you) that without food or water, bonking is inevitable. So the pros live by the code of religious eating and drinking. It is a part of their riding as much as breathing, and it should be for you, too.

Ignore your buddy who brags that he only needs one bottle for a 4-hour ride in 100-degree heat. Smile kindly on your friend who leaves for your all-day pedaling adventure with a single energy bar. Hero is something you earn when they're on the side of the road, bent over their handlebars unable to go another pedal stroke, and you share your food or water. Because you came prepared, you have some to spare.

Eating vs. Drinking Your Calories

There are two ways to get calories for fuel on the bike. One is eating, the other is drinking. New studies show that the best way to keep a steady intake of calories and hydration into your system is to keep your drink low in calories (which makes it trickier for your body to absorb the fluid) and, as much as possible, eat real food.

When you're on the bike, you lose water and salt through sweat, and as that water transfers to your skin, your blood becomes thicker—which makes it harder for the blood to deliver what the muscles need. So to balance that out, you need to get water back into the system. In the meantime, your muscles and skin are battling for bloodflow—your skin to get rid of heat, and your muscles to keep riding. The more hydrated you are, the less severe this battle gets. In the end, if you don't drink, your skin will always win the battle because being overheated will kill you, so your body will default to taking care of you by sweating. This is one way the dreaded bonk will set in.

Although it may seem like a great idea to get your calories and electrolytes through your drink, the problem is that many sports drinks made to use on the bike are too concentrated and focused on giving you calories, so they actually draw water out of your bloodstream to

Recipes to Help Fuel Yourself

HERE ARE A FEW RECIPES AND IDEAS FOR foods and bars to make at home and eat on the bike. This is a great way to both save money and customize your ride food to your own tastes. Also, it's a great way to get your family involved. You can make them together (or see if they'd be nice enough to make them for you!).

D. Sharp's Energy Bars

(Makes approximately 18 bars)

2	cups rolled oats (can sub a cup of spelt or other rolled grains instead)
1⅓	lb Medjool dates
½	cup chopped almonds (roasted, salted, or raw)
½	cup roasted/salted pecan pieces
1	cup large hazelnuts, chopped or bashed
3–5	Tbsp agave or maple syrup
½	cup coconut flakes, dried fruits such as cherries or raisins, seeds like chia or sesame, chocolate chips, or any other additions you crave

Preheat oven to 325 degrees Fahrenheit. Spread oats on a baking sheet and toast for 15 minutes, stirring once halfway through.

Chop dates into ¼-inch pieces. Chop nuts. When the oats are toasted, mix nuts, oats, and dates together in a large bowl. Add any dried fruit or your favorite fun additions.

Add syrup, starting with 3 tablespoons and adding more as needed until the mixture can be easily pressed together by hand and will hold together as a large ball.

Press ball into a well-greased or parchment-lined 7 x 11-inch baking dish, or in the corner of a greased or lined baking sheet until it is a rectangle ¾-inch in depth. Bake for 20 minutes. Cut into 1 x 2-inch bars.

Store in a sealed, dry place. Wrap each bar in plastic wrap or parchment paper to easily carry in your jersey pocket on the ride.

Nutritional Value: Per bar: 230 calories, 9g fat, 40g carb, 5g fiber, 2.5g protein

Stacy Sims Granola Clusters

A wee snack pack that rocks in the pocket ...

1¼	cup rolled oats
⅓	cup chopped almonds or walnuts or sunflower seeds
⅓	cup raw cashews or pistachios
1	Tbsp vanilla bean powder
¼	tsp cinnamon
1¼	oz dried cranberries or raisins

In a heavy-bottom skillet, dry-roast the oats, nuts, vanilla, and cinnamon over low to moderate heat (watch and stir continuously, as it can burn quickly!). When toasty, transfer to a glass bowl and stir in dried fruit with 2 tablespoons brown rice syrup. Mix well until coated.

Spread onto a cookie sheet to cool. Break into clusters.

Dr. Stacy Sims Protein Power Bites
(Makes about 23 1-inch balls)

½	cup vanilla protein powder (can be vegan or dairy)
¾	cup natural chunky almond or peanut butter
¼	cup nonfat dried milk
¼	cup brown rice syrup
¼	tsp ground cinnamon
1	tsp espresso powder (optional)
1	Tbsp ground flaxseed
2	Tbsp unsweetened Dutch processed cocoa powder or coconut or almond meal (for rolling)

Combine all ingredients (except cocoa/coconut meal/almond meal) in a large prep bowl and mix until thoroughly combined. Place dough in fridge for 20 to 30 minutes, until it hardens up a bit.

Roll into bite-sized balls (you can use a melon cuber). Roll formed balls in cocoa powder or coconut or almond meal to coat.

Store in an airtight container in the fridge. When ready to use, put them in a sandwich baggie in your pocket.

Nutritional Value: Per ball: 80 calories, 4g fat, 5g carb, 5g protein

Rice Crispy Re-do

Make good old rice crispy bars (with marshmallows and cereal), but add 4 tablespoons of nut butter before completely melting the marshmallows.

digest—even if they are in a solution of water. This can cause stomach cramping and bloating, not to mention dehydration.

The solution is to get the majority of your calories from food, and keep your fluids to a source that has some electrolytes but not too many carbs. Another benefit from separating the two is that on hotter days, you'll need more fluid, but not necessarily more calories. Keeping the two in their own categories lets you regulate each as you need.

Fueling in the Saddle

Your body already knows how to digest food well, so when someone says, "I can't eat on the bike!" you know that's just plain silly. You already eat at least three times a day, right? On the bike, your main priority is to keep a good input of carbs going. On longer rides, throwing in a little fat or protein is good, too. The general guideline for what to eat and when to eat it starts after the first hour of your ride. In other words, if you're riding only an hour or a little over, you don't need to eat (but you always need to drink). If you plan on riding over 2 hours, you should start eating 45 minutes to an hour into your ride, and keep eating small amounts every 15 to 20 minutes.

Overall, you need around 30 to 60 grams of carbs an hour, or about 3 to 4 calories per kilogram per hour of food, for a moderate ride. To give you some reference, one medium banana is around 30 grams of carbs and 120 calories. Spread out your eating into 15- to 20-minute intervals over the hour. Remember, your blood is already working to keep your muscles fueled and your body temperature down. If you eat the whole banana at once, it will force more of your blood to concentrate in your digestive system, pulling it away from the more important jobs it needs to do to keep you going.

It's also harder for your body to digest a large amount of calories at once as opposed to small amounts. The trick to not running out of fuel is to keep eating small amounts of food every 15 to 20 minutes on your ride. Think of how you feel after a big Thanksgiving meal versus a small afternoon snack. When riders claim to not be able to eat on the bike, it's usually because they're trying to eat too much at once instead of spacing it out into small snack bites. "But I'm not hungry!" you insist. If you wait until you feel hunger, you're already in too much of a deficit to catch up—and you'll be behind for the rest of your ride.

To keep yourself honest, use your bike computer or watch to set a timer to go off every 20 minutes. Do not play the "promises" game, where you know you should grab food from your pocket but are going to wait until "the next intersection," "the top of the climb," "when we slow down," or "at mile forty." If it's time to eat, eat. No compromises.

To find foods that work on the bike, look at what your body needs and how much space you have to carry it. Food needs to be able to fit in your pocket, be easily grabbed and manipulated with one hand, and have a high concentration of easily absorbed carbohydrates. Oh, and most importantly, it should be food that tastes good so you'll *want* to eat it.

Choosing real, natural food is a good place to start. High-carb foods that transport well on the bike include bananas, nuts, peanut butter and honey sandwiches cut into quarters, or snack bars made with rice or quinoa—which are great if you want to switch from sweet to savory. It helps if it has fat or proteins, but the majority of your calories should be coming from carbohydrates. One thing to be aware of is to not take in too much fresh or dried fruit, or other high-fiber foods. These take more energy to digest, and can cause an upset stomach.

Real food not only tastes great, but it's also much cheaper than energy bars and gels. These are also good things to have on hand, but it's best not to count on them for all your calories. Energy bars are very calorie-dense, so it's easy to eat too many or too much. Gels, goos, and chews are okay if you're bonking or near the end of a ride that is over 3 or 4 hours—like a century or a bike tour—and you need a little energy but don't feel like eating more food. But always remember that you need to drink lots of water with them if you want to avoid gut rot and dehydration. A better and more easily digested boost can come from foods you can find at the gas station (like gummy bears or jelly beans) or glucose tablets, which don't take as much water from your system to digest. These are also great for racing where you're trying to be as light and compact as possible, and when you may not have time to grab your food.

If you haven't already practiced, it's good to get in the habit of being able to reach into your jersey pocket while riding with one hand on your handlebars to grab and eat your food. You don't want to stop every 15 to 20 minutes to eat. Find a parking lot or quiet street and practice grabbing, opening, and closing your food packaging and putting any leftovers or garbage back into your pocket while on the move. Concentrate on holding your line and not wavering from your position in the road. After a while, you'll know how much speed you need to hold to smoothly grab a bite as you roll, and eating while you ride will become second nature.

Drinking and Riding

We've already talked a lot about how important hydration is and that even on the shortest rides you need to drink. First, get into the good habit of regularly reaching for your water bottle. You need to take in around one to two 16-ounce bottles of fluid an hour, no matter how long you're on the bike. Like food, it's hard for your body to take it all in at once, so it's better spaced out over 10-minute intervals. Drink 3 to 4 ounces at a time—that's a few big glugs, not sips.

If you don't feel comfortable reaching down for your water bottle yet, spend a whole afternoon just practicing reaching down for it, taking a drink and returning the bottle to its cage. Sometimes this is harder than it looks, so investing an afternoon that you would be out pedaling to learning this small skill is huge if you're going to have a good ride without getting dehydrated.

Again, hydrating is something that most nonprofessional cyclists forget to do all the time, so get in the habit by setting an alarm or watching the clock. After working on this regularly over weeks and months, your body will start to feel a little thirsty every 10 minutes without the reminders. If it's hot out, aim for two bottles of water or an electrolyte drink an hour. No matter what, you cannot catch up if you get dehydrated. In fact, even if you follow this guide to the letter, you'll still end up a little dehydrated at the end of the ride, as it's impossible to keep up with what your body will use.

Caffeine: Friend or Foe?

Most of us have some kind of relationship with caffeine. Whether it's a few cups of coffee to get your morning rolling or a simple cup of green or black tea, it's a ritual we'd be loath to give up.

Lucky for us, caffeine has been proven to be an excellent performance booster on the bike as well. Beyond making you more alert and focused, it can help you burn carbs a little faster and stimulate the release of fatty acids, which help you save on your glycogen stores while still staying fueled.

It was thought for years that caffeine was to be avoided because it would dehydrate you—especially bad on hot days. Finally, a scientist thought to study it and found that it doesn't make you sweat or pee any more than any other drink. It does, however, improve your strength, endurance, and perception of how hard you're pushing—meaning you can go harder with less pain. The benefits last even after your workout is over, as it can also decrease post-ride soreness.

That being said, even if you consider yourself a regular coffee addict, you might want to cut back a little to conserve your boost. If you start your ride stimulated, not only will you make yourself jittery and anxious, but you also won't be able to get the boost you need at the end of the ride when you may be hurting. Professional and amateur cyclists agree on one thing: In the last quarter of your ride, an icy cola on a hot day or a hot espresso on a cold one can be a game changer, turning your ride from a death march to a dance home. If you don't have access to a store or café, a caffeinated gel or chew can do the trick—though it's definitely not as tasty.

CHAPTER 34

Post-Ride Recovery: Slow Down, Take It Easy

HOW YOU TREAT YOURSELF AFTER A RIDE IS JUST AS IMPOR-
tant as what you eat before or during your ride. For many riders who get the cycling
bug, it becomes a frequent or even daily routine to have a ride be part of your day. So
it's important when you get off the bike to take care of yourself so you're ready to roll
the day after, or the day after that. Proper recovery also helps you make the most of
all the effort you put into the bike today. When you skip this step, your body has a
harder time completely building from the hours of work you put in.

If you've been cruising only for an hour or two, this isn't as critical. When you've
been on the bike longer, or if your ride has been intense, eating for recovery can triple
the rate at which your muscles repair and restock their supplies of glycogen. There are
two windows to pay attention to, and the first is the most acute. You have 20 to 30
minutes to get some protein and a few carbs in your system, before the benefits start
falling off. It's often called a "glycogen window" because it's only open for so long,
then slams shut.

Carbohydrates Plus Protein Speeds Recovery

Dr. Sims advises, "You have thirty minutes or less after riding to maximize protein intake for muscle synthesis, and up to two hours for glycogen recovery. The addition of protein to carbohydrates post-exercise increases glycogen recovery more so than just carbs alone; but the addition of protein supercharges recovery.

"Research also shows that combining protein with carbohydrates within thirty minutes of exercise nearly doubles the insulin response, which results in more stored glycogen. The optimal carbohydrate-to-protein ratio for this effect is 4:1 (four grams of carbohydrates for every one gram of protein). One study found that athletes who refueled with carbohydrates and protein had one hundred percent greater muscle glyco-gen stores than those who only ate carbohydrates. Insulin was also highest in those who consumed a carbohydrate and protein drink."

In this period, it's time to reward yourself for all your hard work. Chocolate milk has been proven in studies to be a great recovery drink, and one beer has the right amount of carbs—though you want to still add in some protein to hit the right balance. Smoothies are particularly good. You can throw in yogurt, milk (or a milk alternative like almond), banana, honey, frozen fruit—even a little squirt of chocolate syrup never hurt anybody. Studies have also found a small amount of caffeine aids in recovery as well, so a cup of green tea or a half-shot of espresso can help, too.

Whatever you do, your immediate recovery usually isn't a full meal. It's a high-carb, low-protein boost to get your body in build-and-repair

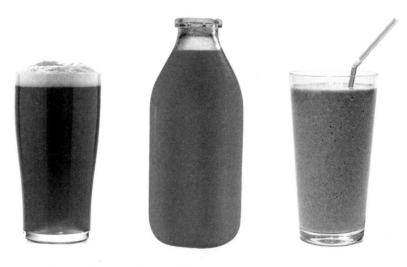

Recovering from your workout can be as rewarding as drinking a beer, chocolate milk, or a smoothie.

Protein is the Post-Exercise Powerhouse

CONSUMING PROTEIN HAS OTHER IMPORTANT USES AFTER exercise. Protein provides the amino acids necessary to rebuild muscle tissue that is damaged during intense, prolonged exercise. It can also increase the absorption of water from the intestines and improve muscle hydration. The amino acids in protein can also stimulate the immune system, making you more resistant to colds and other infections.

—DR. STACY SIMS, exercise physiologist and nutrition scientist of thermoregulation, hydration, and performance nutrition

mode and give you a chance to take off your cycling gear, clean up your bike, and hit the shower. After that, try to get a full meal within 2 hours of being off the bike. Don't overeat even if you did have a long ride. If you were following our advice in "Fueling in the Saddle," on page 183, you should have taken in enough calories that you don't have to stuff yourself after the ride.

CHAPTER 35

Getting Lean: Using Your Bike to Shrink Your Waistline

THE BIKE IS A GREAT WAY TO GET LEAN. IF YOU'RE NOT ALREADY fit or athletic, you'll likely find that you'll shed a few pounds as you go farther and farther on your bicycle. However, some people find that they *gain* weight when they start cycling. How could this be?

There are a few reasons. The most common is the reward system. Hey, you worked hard on the bike today, so maybe you have an extra cookie or two, or one more beer at the end of the night. But it's a delicate balance between losing weight and treating yourself. Don't overcompensate.

At the other end of the spectrum, there are the riders who cut their calories way back and hope to see the pounds magically melt away. Unfortunately, our bodies have a built-in safety system to keep us alive as long as possible. If you drop your calorie intake too much or too suddenly—especially when you're exercising—your body goes into a panic and will try to conserve as many calories as possible to keep you from starving. Instead of burning calories, your body will be saving them.

The best way to shed a few pounds is to figure out how much on average your body can burn from cycling, and then take in just slightly fewer calories than that number. This can be challenging because you need fuel before you ride, fuel on the ride, and fuel to recover. To really be successful, you need to pay close attention to portions and trade out any bad eating habits—like too much processed food or sugar—for eating healthy, real foods rich in nutrients and the right kinds of fuels.

Take these tips from Dr. Sims. "The body is primed for carbohydrate consumption in the morning and becomes more sensitive as the day wears on. Protein becomes the goer in the afternoon and evening as most reparation occurs during sleep. To maximize the body's natural hormonal rhythms, think of eating complex carbs with a bit of protein in the morning, combination at lunch, and more protein orientation with veggies and a bit of fresh fruit toward the evening."

Some will find that they shed some pounds right off the bat, but eventually we're all faced with this tipping point and when we get there, we have to either decide to love our bodies for all the wonderful things they can already do for us, or knuckle down, pay attention, and concentrate on getting lean. Neither one is right or wrong, good or bad. It's up to your priorities and goals, not only when you're on the bike, but just as much when you're off it.

PART IX

TRAINING: TUNING YOUR BODY AND YOUR MIND

There is a thought out there that to ride bikes, you must get serious, and to get serious, you must train. This contains both truth and total nonsense.

You can be serious about cycling—even cycling every day—and never, ever train. If you plan on sticking to commuting, bike touring, recreational rides, and hanging out in your usual spot in your pack of friends on a group ride, then you can be perfectly happy never training. Simply riding your bike will be more than enough. You can even improve—get faster, lose weight, become more efficient—without ever formally training. This is especially true for beginner cyclists who have plenty of other things to concentrate on, like riding skills and technique.

Cycling makes your body a better tuned, fitter machine. The more you ride, the more your body adapts to being efficient in its use of oxygen. Over time, as you cycle, you grow more capillaries in your muscles as a response to their hunger for more fuel. Your body gets more efficient at optimizing the fuel you have to burn. Your heart gets stronger, making it better at pumping the blood and oxygen to where it's needed, while your body produces more enzymes that help that oxygen burn more fat. This is what makes the hill easier and easier to climb—a little less heart pounding, chest squeezing, and muscle burning.

However, with that being said, you can get only so far without training that specifically targets the adaptations your body can make (like endurance, climbing, or speed). You will hit walls where you can't ride any faster, gain more endurance, or get any stronger climbing, when your results in a local century ride stagnate to the same times year after year. For some riders this might happen over a season; for others it might take years. It's common to blame this on "getting older," but for most people that's just another excuse.

The question to ask yourself is, do you really need to adapt further? For many riders, being on the bike isn't about going faster or attacking harder—it's about enjoying the ride. This is a beautiful, wonderful, lovely concept that has brought people onto the saddle and kept them there for lifetimes. Simply being on the bike and reveling in the fun, freedom, and regular fitness you experience is more than enough for most riders.

However, if you're someone who likes formal goals or who wants to race, is very competitive, likes structure, and wants to push your body to new levels, then training might be just the ticket for you.

CHAPTER 36

Tuning Your Body

FIRST LET'S TALK ABOUT WHAT TRAINING IS AND ISN'T. FOR many beginner riders, the simple act of riding a bike may seem like training. It's true that getting out and spinning the pedals—however hard or fast or leisurely—is indeed exercising, but it's not really training. Other new riders think it means pushing yourself as far and hard as you possibly can every time you ride. This is a speedy way to get injured or burn out, fast, and it's not training either. Beginner riders also tend to frame the idea of training with fitness, but most times you're on the bike you're contributing to your well-being. Training is a lot more involved than just staying fit.

Training, at its root, means focusing, planning, and paying attention to specifically target-building your body's ability to adapt. At the top, professional riders are training all the time—literally. When a rider decides to go pro, it's a little like deciding to sign your life over to someone else. During their season (which runs between 10 and 11 months of the year), professional riders will have coaches, doctors, nutritionists, physiologists, and an entire staff of people telling them exactly what to do each day.

"Okay, so they have to go ride their bikes all day," you think. "That doesn't sound like such a big deal." But for them, training not only dictates their riding and how that time is spent on the bike. It also touches every other part of their life as well, including how much to eat and when, how much to sleep and when, how much to walk or do any other movement off the bike and when to do it—down to each calorie and minute of shut-eye and weigh-in on the scale, down to the days and minutes riders will officially be "off." Yes, this also includes their romantic and personal lives. There is no such thing as leaving work at the end of the day because their job is 24 hours day, 7 days a week, and affects every facet of their lives. Training at this level is a total life commitment, because it is a career where the workers are attempting to be at the absolute top of their field and concentrating every part of their day toward that goal.

Thankfully, training for the amateur cyclist is a lot easier, because it mainly involves following a plan only for your time on the bike, with a little tweaking of your life here and there. You get to decide what time of day you'll do it and how you'll spend the rest of your day around it, including what, how much, and when to eat, drink, and sleep—though there are recommendations on how to maximize those, too.

In the end, a training plan is designed to tune your body for a certain end goal. That can be as vague as "becoming a stronger climber" or as specific as getting your best result at a particular race or ride. Either way, it's a concentrated effort to improve that is scientifically structured for you to succeed. Working toward a goal and meeting it can be one of the most satisfying feelings in the world.

If you follow a training plan, you will see improvements and get results. Every day you'll be extra motivated to ride because your mindset will switch from thinking about what kind of ride you want—or if you even want to ride that day—to checking in on what's on the schedule. Following a plan also gives you the chance to fully flesh out what success will look like for you, which is very helpful for achieving your goals. Off the bat, you know that there is a beginning, middle, and end to what you're doing. It's an adventure to tick off your highs and lows of how each week (and your body) shapes up and a countdown until the big day arrives.

Riding Hard vs. Riding Smart

When you were a kid racing your friends through the neighborhood, it was easy to see how to get faster—just grow a few inches and always pedal harder. As adults who have bigger goals, the childhood "pedal harder" method is pretty much a bust. But many people cling to it as a sure thing while never really hitting their full potential, which sounds a little backward. How can pushing hard keep you from attaining better results?

Much like nutrition, it's all about quality over quantity. Over the years, physiologists have spent countless hours studying what can optimize your body's output to get the best results. They have found that there are times to put the pedal to the metal, to go steady, or to soft-pedal and enjoy the day. Sometimes getting off the bike—or picking a different activity altogether—makes you stronger in the saddle overall.

This often involves daily, weekly, and monthly cycles with periods of stress, rest, and then allowing your body to adapt. To rebuild, your body must have periods of low stress—whether that's physical or mental. Rest and exertion must each be held in a delicate balance, and in training both hold equal weight.

This is common throughout every training cycle. In a given ride, you may stress then rest. Most weeks, you'll have stress days, easy days, and rest days. Monthly, you'll have 3 weeks of building through progressively challenging workouts, then a week of easy pedaling to allow your body to rebuild.

Half of the work is pushing yourself, and the other half is letting yourself recover. How is recovery work? The number one way most riders sabotage their training is by doing too much. On a day you feel fresh and frisky, it will be challenging to go slow or not ride at all. If you're sick or life gets in the way of your training plan, you'll want to go harder to make up for it. Both of these are easy traps to avoid if you remember that going harder than your workout recommends is almost never helpful. Respect that your body needs quality time to repair and build, so you can hit your next goal even stronger.

Your long-term training will likely happen in seasonal cycles as well. You might follow an 8- or 12-week plan, hit your mark, then decide to take some time off from training before setting off toward the next goal. Some people only train once a year, others love it so much they train year-round—of course, with a few select months of rest.

Getting in the Zone

Beyond tracking your efforts, you'll also need to follow a structured training plan. We've talked about the rest and rebuild cycles and how to track your efforts. To put them together, you have to aim your efforts into particular zones for designated amounts of time during your ride. These zones are the first part of the building blocks that will help you to optimize your rides if you're using them as workouts toward particular targets.

In most training plans, your daily workout is divided into either a description of a zone or some technical training terms. Here's how they break down.

RECOVERY: This is the pace you should be at on rest or easy days. This is a breezy, unchallenging pace that most riders have a hard time staying in because it's *that* slow. It might involve very light pedaling and a lot of coasting. Recovery gives your body a chance to rebuild.

ENDURANCE: This is a pace you could cruise along at for a whole ride without hurrying. Your body is getting into an aerobic intensity, but it's never a ride you'd describe as hard or challenging. This is the effort you could do for a long haul while holding a conversation. This is the "fat burning" zone, though you'll burn more when you combine it with harder efforts.

TEMPO: A somewhat hard effort. Like going from a slow jam to rocking out, you're picking it up a bit. Your heart is starting to beat faster, but it's a little more stilted. You don't feel like you're going too fast, but just a little harder than you'd normally feel comfortable cruising along at. You couldn't hold this pace forever, but you could for a while—similar to how you might feel on a long, not very steep climb, or if you were riding with someone who was just a little bit faster than you. This pace helps you grow your aerobic capacity, which is the base on which you get stronger and faster.

RACE PACE: Even if you don't race, this is how fast you'd go if you did. This is what you think of when someone says "go hard." This is a focused, intense effort during which you should start to feel your legs burning and you're reaching the edge of what your body can do for any length of time. You won't be able to talk much, if at all, at race pace. Afterward you feel glad you backed off. Just like tempo builds a base, this expands your body's capacity to make accelerations and hold on when the riding gets fast.

MAX EFFORT: This is the all-out effort. You won't be at this pace for very long (usually 10 to 15 seconds) because it works best when done in very short bursts. While there you'll be sucking in air, your heart will be pounding, and you'll likely be in what cyclists describe as a "pain cave." Thankfully, not only is it quick, but you also get a lot of bang for your buck. These efforts help you burn fat, build muscle, and increase power and speed.

Training Zones

BECAUSE HEART RATE IS NOT ALWAYS reliable, it's best to use it with your perceived rate of exertion.

TRAINING ZONE	% OF MAX HEART RATE	PERCEIVED RATE OF EXERTION
Zone 1: Recovery	60–65%	1–2
Zone 2: Endurance	66–75%	3–4
Zone 3: Tempo	76–82%	5–6
Zone 4: Race Pace	83–89%	7–8
Zone 5: Max Effort	90–94%	9–10

CHAPTER 37

Tracking Your Efforts

DEPENDING ON YOUR FOCUS, THERE ARE MANY DIFFERENT types of training that vary in duration and effort. They all involve structuring a defined plan for the stress/rest model, which basically tells you which zones of exertion—or how hard you should go—you should be in and for how long. But how do you keep track of how hard you're pushing your body and when you need to rest?

Rating of Perceived Exertion: The Big RPE!

If you're in pain and you find yourself at the doctor's office, they've created an easy and fairly accurate scale to learn how severe it is, simply by asking you how bad you feel on a scale of 1 to 10. The RPE (rating of perceived exertion) system is based on exactly the same concept. It's the easiest (and most affordable) way to keep tabs on how hard you're working because your own judgment of how hard it is *for you* is nearly as accurate as most of the other methods we'll talk about. The downside is it only works if it's used correctly, which is sometimes hard to do with consistency.

We have a hard time being truthful to ourselves if we have ulterior motives. When you eat that doughnut for breakfast but you're supposed to have an easy day on the bike, wanting to work off those calories might sabotage your soft-pedaling. If you just had a fight with your boyfriend or girlfriend, it might be harder to concentrate and keep up the entire 15 minutes of high intensity you're supposed to put out. In the end, having some of the more high-tech gadgets that give you hard numbers as you pedal can help keep you honest on both easy and hard days.

However, those can be an investment of both time and money, so the RPE scale is a great choice for most new cyclists who are just getting into training for the first time. The scale looks like this:

1–2: **Easy.** Sitting on the couch watching Netflix. You should be breathing normally, completely relaxed.

3–5: **Not hard.** Getting up off the couch and going for a walk—maybe even speed-walking. Your breathing is a little faster, but you can easily have a conversation in which you don't have to take a breath until the end of the sentence.

6–8: **Putting in the effort.** Taking it up to a jog or, if you're feeling frisky, a run. You might be able to talk in phrases, but your breaths are short, hard, and fast enough that holding a conversation would be a challenge.

9–10: **Maxing it out.** Running fast to running a sprint as if your life depends on it. No air for talking, you're using it all to keep your body moving—to the point you might even be gasping for air.

Heart Rate

The second most common and effective way of keeping track of your intensity level is using a heart-rate monitor. This little gadget works in conjunction with either a band on your wrist or around your chest that measures the electronic pulses of your heart in beats per minute (bpm), then sends them wirelessly to a monitor on your bike so you can keep an eye on what's happening in your body. The most affordable of these are separate from your cycling computer that tracks your mileage, speed, time, or cadence, so you'll have to find more room on your handlebars for another gadget, or pay extra for a computer that does all of these things in one package.

It will involve a little more math to get started. You have to use easy formulas to get some baseline stats for how many bpm your body needs to hit to be in a particular zone of effort. Keeping track of your heart rate can also lead to wanting to use software or websites to really track your results, since you'll have concrete numbers to plug in. In other words, using heart rate is a great fit if you're the type of person who likes to geek out a bit.

So, first off, you'll want to figure out your *maximum heart rate* (MHR), which is the absolute highest number of beats your heart can kick out in 1 minute. All the other training zones are based off of this magic number, and it will differ for everyone based on age and fitness level. The easiest and quickest formula for figuring it out is 208 − 0.7(your age). For example, for a 32-year-old man it would be 208 − 0.7(32) = 185.6 bpm. Note that this is a general formula, and there are others that work very similarly. Usually the results for each person will be within about 5 bpm of one another, so your zones will be close no matter the calculation you choose.

The most accurate way to find your max is by testing it on the bike—which is best done under the supervision of a trainer and with the green light from your doctor, and is the most accu-

rate when you're starting a training program. This is a good choice if you're already very fit, because being in shape heavily influences your heart rate.

Although this is more accurate than just RPE, the best way to monitor your intensity is by combining your heart rate with your RPE. Together they can keep you in touch with whether you're hitting the zone you're aiming for. Your heart rate is also easily influenced— by caffeine, stress, adrenaline, and getting enough sleep. Whether you're testing your MHR on the bike or trying to figure out if you're hitting your targets on a workout, take into

How Much Effort Should You Put Into Finding Your Effort?

HERE'S A SIMPLE GRAPH ON HOW INVESTED you might be in tracking your efforts during workouts. The more you spend, the more accurate your numbers will be—but that comes at a larger investment of both time and money.

Perceived Rate of Exertion: x = 10 min, y = $0
Online Software: x = 30 min, y = $0–$25
Heart-Rate Monitors: x= 1 hr, y= $50–$500
Power Monitors: x= 1–3 hours, y= $1,500–$3,000

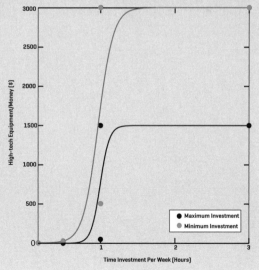

account any extenuating circumstances that might influence it. For example, if you downed that double espresso before heading out for your ride, your heart rate might be sky-high, but your RPE low. Use your noggin—you know better than any trainer or formula if you're hitting your goals for the ride.

Power Meters

This is the method of the pros and hard-core athletes—or other riders who want to invest heavily in their training methods. No way around it, power meters are expensive, starting at around $1,600 for the cheapest model (because some of them also need a special wheel or crank set to be installed). This device measures the watts—or power—the rider puts out. This is the cleanest, clearest, and most dependable method for measuring workload on the bike.

Power meters don't lie, they don't fluctuate, and they can't be influenced by other factors. You either hit your wattage goals, or you don't.

However, to read it and use the numbers it provides, you also need to micro-monitor how your power varies on hills, flats, in the wind, and when riding for speed or endurance. Most athletes who opt for this also have access to software programs that allow them to upload their workouts so their professional trainers can follow every moment. These trainers are also likely to set up their training plans for them and monitor their numbers. If heart rate is the path to maximizing your effort, following your wattage is like getting a degree in your own fitness. Since this is beyond what most beginners need, it likely will be overkill for you. If you're intrigued, talk with a professional trainer or coach about your options and how to get started using power meters.

CHAPTER 38

Finding a Training Plan

NOW THAT YOU HAVE ALL THE INFO YOU NEED TO TRACK YOUR efforts, it's time to find something to do with it. If you've gotten this far, you're interested enough to invest some serious time and effort. Your next step is to decide how much money you want to invest and how specific you need to be with your program to reach your goals. If you just want to get a little stronger on the bike overall or climb faster, you probably could do well with a book, website, or magazine. On the other hand, if your goals are to slim down or win the big Fourth of July criterium in your hometown, you might want to consider a coach.

Online

In this day and age, we're connected more than ever electronically. Websites and training apps on smartphones are affordable and can give you generic, comprehensive plans or individual workouts. This can be fun and interactive, as some apps are made to sync up to your computer or heart-rate monitor and will load up your daily or weekly totals for you. The downside is that if you have questions about your numbers or what the workouts mean, you're going to have to try to research that yourself to find the answers you're looking for. Although it's a great way to get straightforward, easy-to-follow advice, since there are so many voices chiming in it can be difficult to wade through and know who and what is the best to follow. Bicycling.com is a great place to start if you're looking for some simple workouts or training plans, and it has plenty of articles to answer most questions you might have.

Magazines

Magazines are another great resource because all the material you need is in print, so it's easier to sit down with and absorb the content. The beauty of most publications is that they offer information on that month's theme, so you're likely to find more information than just a plan—you'll also find the details on why and how it works. Magazines can give you a chance to better educate yourself about what the possibilities are so you can make a well-informed decision on what's best for you. Along with the website, *Bicycling* magazine features regular articles on how to train, including specific training plans, fitness tips, and more.

Books

If you like magazines, books can be an even better choice because they tend to offer long-range cycling plans and provide more specific information. This is a great way to immerse yourself in the culture and science behind training. You can expect expert advice that delves into the finer points of what you're hoping to accomplish. Books are also more specific—you may want to lose weight but are short on time—so they help raise your chances of your training being successful.

Many of *Bicycling* magazine's regular contributors—such as Selene Yeager, Chris Carmichael, and Ben Hewitt, all of whom have worked with professional athletes and beginner cyclists alike—have written books on how to go about training.

Coaching

Having a professional to talk over your goals, formulate a plan, and check in with on a regular basis is the ultimate in both formulating and executing your training plan. A professional coach has the expertise to read your data, analyze your stats, and adjust your workouts to best meet your needs. A coach can also give you the most valuable thing a developing rider needs—feedback. Of course, this comes at a price. Hiring a coach is the biggest investment when it comes to training. Like a gym membership, most coaches or coaching programs offer different plans priced at different levels depending on personalization and the amount the coach will have contact with you. The more attention and specification you have, the more it will cost. This can vary from, at minimum, only e-mail or phone contact to the coach actually going for a ride with you and giving you a daily or weekly evaluation of your numbers.

Another advantage of coaches is having accountability. It's easy for any of us to skip a day of riding or get off our program if we're the only ones keeping ourselves honest. Having someone else to report to—especially when you're paying good money for his or her expertise—is that little nudge to keep you going and motivated, even on days when the weather is bad or you don't feel so hot.

Taking It Inside

When you get to the point where you want to be pedaling year-round, this means heading indoors. Whether it's the sweltering summers of the Southwest or the brutal winters in the north, long days at work or a life packed with your family's schedule, there will be days—especially if you're on a training plan—when riding outside is simply not an option.

Riding indoors is convenient, but hard and sometimes rather boring. The lack of coasting, cruising, or tailwinds makes your effort that much harder—which is good actually, because you can focus the intensity of your ride and still get great results. If you love to watch your numbers—like heart rate or speed—indoor cycling is free of other distractions like traffic or suicidal squirrels.

If you already belong to a gym, you can join one of their *spin classes*. This is a great opportunity to work on your pedaling technique and use some very nice indoor bikes with more computer bells and whistles. It also has the bonus of a professional teacher guiding a class through a specific workout aimed at speed, climbing, or power on the bike—like having a coach for a day. Riders often find that with this little extra focus, their riding improves more inside than it does outside.

If sticking close to home is a better option, *stationary trainers* are an affordable option (they cost about the same as a 3-month gym membership). The downside is that you lose the group aspect of the class as well as the teacher. The upside is that you can specifically dial in the workout you want to do—and when you want to do it. It's also good to plan on setting

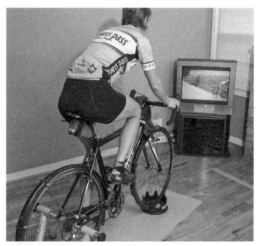

A stationary trainer can be a great way to keep riding your bicycle year-round.

your trainer up somewhere cool (possibly with a fan directed at you) and with some kind of entertainment, like a video or podcast.

Stationary trainers attach to your rear wheel, creating a stable platform so you can easily stay upright without having to balance. They come in three basic types.

Wind trainers are the loudest and most inexpensive, but they are pretty realistic when compared to riding outside on the road in terms of pedaling resistance. Your back tire spins a roller attached to a fan that provides more resistance the faster you go.

Magnetic trainers are in the same price range as wind ones, but are quieter. Also, when you pedal faster, your resistance doesn't get harder, which makes hitting your workout numbers tough. Some come with resistance adjustments to try to overcome this flaw.

Fluid trainers are the most expensive, but for your dollar you get the quietest and most realistic road experience. One problem on older models was that the oil inside—which provided the resistance—would leak. Most current models have overcome this problem, but be wary of buying a used one.

CHAPTER 39

Tuning Your Life: Finding Time to Ride, Cross-Training, and Life/Bike Balance

WE'VE TALKED ABOUT TRAINING AS BEING A PATTERN OF stress and rebuilding, but your life is actually the same way. If you aren't balanced in terms of how you fit cycling into your life, you're not going to get stronger, faster, or healthier, or (worst of all) have much fun.

The truth of road cycling is that it takes time—not just in the sense of months or years, but in the hours. There isn't really such a thing as a quick, 20-minute training ride. Unless you're commuting or not as concerned with gaining fitness, you have to put in a minimum of an hour per ride (usually closer to an hour and a half and up to as much as 3 hours).

Riding that much can be a fun escape, but eventually the same routes will become monotonous, and all that time on the bike can even lead to injury. It's also a good idea to add in fun alternatives off the bike that will help shape up the rest of your body (and mind). Some of us need a little extra inspiration to get on the bike, so finding people to ride with who challenge you or an online forum to "race" other cyclists can be motivating.

Of course, with all this activity and your regular, hectic life schedule, it's sometimes a challenge to get enough sleep or to see your friends or family. Making road cycling a part of your life should never mean sacrificing quality in other areas, so here are some tips on how to integrate your new road cycling interest into your already busy life.

Carving Out Time to Ride

The most common pitfall to regularly getting on your bike is finding the time to ride. "My life is hectic enough, how am I supposed to find more time?" cry many new cyclists. There are spaces and ways to find time. Most involve manipulating the little pieces that are already there—most of us are just too busy checking in on social networks (again) to find it.

You likely just invested a good amount of money into your bike and gear, so don't let them languish in your basement. You're going to have to get creative about finding time. It will not magically appear like sunshine breaking through a cloudy day. The first step is to make riding one of your priorities: looking ahead at your week and planning your times to ride. Sit down and take a close look at your daily schedule. Where can you trim? Can you go to bed earlier and start your day a little sooner? Can your commute to work be a part (or all) of your ride?

Making the most of weekends is key. One tip is to prepare your dinners on Sunday evening for the whole week. You'll create more evening time to ride during the week and have lovely, healthy meals to come home to. As for rides, starting early—before your kids or significant other is awake—allows for your ride time and a way to have a great breakfast with your family when you return—bed head meets helmet head. Maybe there's a weekend family picnic you could ride to instead of driving, and your husband can meet you there with a clean change of clothes. If you can, consider investing in a babysitter or hiring the kid next door to mow your lawn. It's a few dollars well spent if you consider riding a part of your mental health as well as your physical well-being.

Once you find the time, write it down on the calendar and stick to the plan—without pushing the start time back or skipping it altogether, both of which can quickly become a bad habit. Keeping a log of your rides—whether that's uploading your cycling computer's data to a program or simply keeping a little ride journal to track your miles and how you felt—will give you a sense of accomplishment and keep you motivated. Always remember: The key to cycling is momentum, and going for rides inspires going for even more rides.

Rise to the Occasion

The quietest time of day is the morning, so take advantage of it. This is when your ride is least likely to be sabotaged by the rest of your life, and it gets checked off your list for the day. Mornings are quiet on the road, so you're also least likely to be hounded by traffic. Guaranteed, you'll also have more energy in the morning than after work.

It's a little harder to be motivated early in the day, but this is where good prep work makes all the difference. The pull of a warm bed or hitting the snooze button one more time is a little less tempting when your riding clothes are laid out, your water bottles are waiting for you in the fridge, and you have a quick, easy breakfast planned to get your blood sugar boosted.

For example, Elise works full time and is the mom of three rambunctious kids under 12 with a husband who is in his residency on his way to becoming a doctor. There's not a lot of extra wiggle room in her day, but most days of the week during her racing season she manages to get up an hour before her kids to ride her trainer. This time not only keeps her sane, but also has helped her create a successful, winning strategy for her local races.

Get to Work

This is where commuting by bike starts to look like a great idea. It gives you the chance to readily add on more miles at the beginning or the end of the day, and you'll also get to work wide awake and in a great mood—making your entire day more productive. To pull this off, it really helps to have a workplace that provides showers and lockers so you can put your damp clothes somewhere other than your desk, but there are a lot of innovative ways to get around this. One is a gym membership so you can use their facilities. If you can't fully shower, use baby wipes or a washcloth and a portable, quick-dry camp towel.

Break Into Your Lunch

Like commuting, this can be a little tricky to execute, but it's worth the effort. It's not only the perfect mid-day pick-me-up, it also feels a bit like you're getting away with something. Remember how great recess was? This can help you capture that feeling again. Ask around to see if your building or local club has a regular ride. It's so much easier to get motivated if you know other people are joining you—and if you've told them you'll be coming.

After-Hours

Although this might seem like the go-to time to get your ride in, remember that you'll have a whole day behind you, so your energy may not be the brightest. You'll also have to contend with traffic, working late, and all the other little things life tends to throw your way—like your kids' schedules or community activities—that can interfere with your two-wheel time. To make the most of it, schedule your time carefully and absolutely stick to it. Finding a riding buddy who can go with you or posting your planned workout somewhere public like social networks can give you accountability so you stick to your plan.

Cross-Training

If you find yourself always wanting to be on the bike, you may have fallen for road cycling pretty hard, which is great, wonderful, exciting, and motivating. However, like the rest of life, your body needs balance. If you find yourself wanting to ride year-round, you might want to take a little time either during your week or seasonally to switch things up a bit. This will not only

refresh your muscles, it's also a much-needed boost for your mind to wrap itself around another activity.

Most importantly, road cycling is an activity that is repetitive and holds your body in essentially the same position for the entire time you're exercising. Which means your legs and butt get a great workout, and everything else . . . well, that just kind of tends to waste away a bit. Moving the focus to all those neglected parts of your body is important if you're cycling 10 or more hours a week.

Weight-Bearing Fitness

One of the great things about cycling is that it's a non-weight-bearing activity, which essentially means it's easy on your joints. This is a good thing if you're recovering from an injury. However, without bearing weight on your joints during exercise, your bones can actually start to weaken. This is partially caused by all the calcium you're sweating out and partially because impact exercise helps your bones strengthen. Between the two, it's important to add in other exercises that help your bones buck up and keep their density.

This can be as simple as hiking, jogging, a step-aerobics class, circuit training, or even a dance class. Yes, swing dancing can make you a better cyclist. Don't overlook weight lifting as well. High-rep, low-weight lifting for strengthening and toning can do a world of good for not only your legs, but also for those poor arms that are neglected while you're riding.

Yoga, Pilates, and Isometric Exercises

Speaking of neglected, let's talk a moment about your core. These are all your muscles in the middle—in the front, on the sides, and around the back, too. Most of us think of them only in relation to situps or crunches, but those hit only a small portion of your total core muscles. All of these are so much more important than you'd think—especially on the bike, because any strength or power from your legs actually radiates from your core. If your middle is mushy and neglected, it won't really matter how strong your legs are. It's a little like trying to shoot a cannon from a canoe. You're not going to get good results.

Yoga and Pilates not only help you strengthen these muscles—both are based on starting from a strong core—but also give you the added advantage of stretching. This will help stretch, strengthen, and lengthen your muscles and connective fibers after all the hard work you put into riding. These types of exercises often don't seem hard—which doesn't mean they're not working or that you need to seek out an extra hot yoga session or the hardest Pilates class they offer. Feeling sore for 2 days after is not the goal here. Keep this part of your cross-training light, and you'll have great results and be motivated to keep it as part of your routine.

Off-Season

There comes a time of year when the days become too short and the weather too cold to cycle outdoors, so this is a great opportunity to explore. If you still want to brave the outdoors, skiing makes it easy to keep your legs and glutes in shape. Downhill helps keep up your agility, cross-country is a great aerobic workout, and backcountry gives you the best of both worlds. Or slow down a bit and try snowshoeing.

If you don't have as much time, or weak knees or hips are a problem, head to your nearest indoor pool and take the plunge. It's a power workout in both strength and cardio while being easy on your joints. Swimming is one of the best all-around exercises. It strengthens your core; relieves your poor cycling- and computer-hunched shoulders; builds up the little muscles between your ribs that help you balance and steer on the bike; and lengthens your tight hip flexors.

Life/Bicycle Balance: Paying It Forward

At some point you may find yourself falling in love with road cycling. It's a beautiful thing: the freedom; the call of the road; and gaining fitness, confidence, and an eagerness to explore. Although we talked a bit about finding time to ride, it's also worth mentioning how to balance your newfound passion with all the other things in your life you love . . . like your friends, your family, your husband or wife, your kids. Let's face it: Most people have insanely busy lives these days. Add in family and friends and your other hobbies, and it can be really tough to balance them all out.

Here's a common scenario:

It's Friday night and you're ready to relax, already dreaming of your ride tomorrow with your friends. You have a beer, get your chain oiled and tires inflated, and are all ready to roll for the morning. As you head back upstairs, your wife asks, "So what time do you want to head over to Chloe's game tomorrow?" A quick flash and you remember your daughter has her big league final soccer game, and you promised to be the driver.

These conflicts happen all the time, so it's important to have a game plan to make sure that your time on the bike doesn't take over and your friends and family aren't getting the short end of the stick. There is no bigger troublemaker than taking off to leave your significant other saddled with the task of keeping the household running smoothly and taking care of all the details. Not only will he or she feel neglected, it will likely come with a big side serving of resentment, too. Here are a few ways you can make it all work so that cycling isn't something that takes away from the rest of your life, but rather adds to it.

Organize

Organization is the key, and some of us are terrible at it. If you want to fit cycling in, you have to be clear about what your other obligations and responsibilities are—as well as who wants a piece of your time. Sit down and make a list of all the things you have to do (lawn, laundry, cooking for the week), all the things you have scheduled like work or appointments, the people you want to spend time with (your daughter, your best friend who's having a hard time right now), and, finally, your cycling goals. By being able to look at them all, you can get a better sense of what you're up against.

Communicate

Sit down with the other people in your life and ask them what they want or need from you that week. Maybe your husband wants a night out for a date, so it's best if you tell him you were planning on riding after work Thursday night. Talk about when you're available and coordinate so you can be around (maybe after your rides?) to do things together. Ask what you can do to give your partner some free time while you take up the slack. Volunteering to help take care of a bigger part of the household when you do have time will earn you big points and create reciprocity for when you want to train or ride more.

If you've got kids, ask them how they would like to spend time with you. Have them write down a list. Pick an activity or two a week to do with them so they realize that your bike isn't more important than they are. Asking what's important to them and truly listening to your husband, wife, kids, and friends about what they need will go a long way.

On your end, it's very important for the people in your life who care about you to understand why cycling is important to you. Not as a justification for why you're never home, but to give them perspective: Explain why you're a better person—less stressed, happier, healthier, saner—when you get to ride your bike.

Prioritize

Take the list and make some cuts. Your daughter's soccer game should always win over the ride, but maybe you can hit the road early and make it back in time to be superdad and cheer

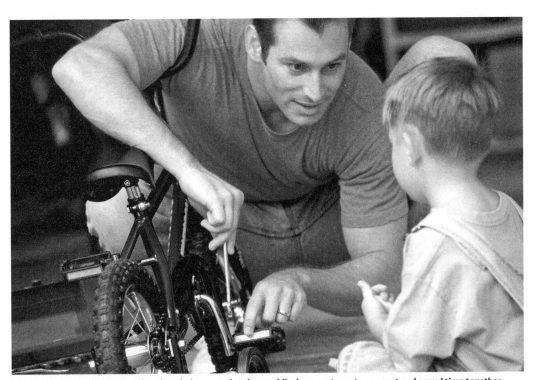

Riding with your family and having them help you maintain your bike is a great way to connect and spend time together.

her on. If the house needs to be cleaned, coordinate with your boyfriend's schedule so you can do it together before you head out on your ride.

Get Them Involved

You have a built-in support crew at your disposal. Maybe your wife would love to try out a new recipe for a nutrition bar (which are nice to snack on at home, too). Your boyfriend doesn't ride? Ask him to go out with you. Bike needs to be cleaned? Teaching your kids about bikes and maintenance is a great way to connect and make them feel like they're a part of that thing that keeps taking you away from them. Get them on their own bikes. If they're not interested, still make an effort to connect with whatever makes them happy.

Take Off and Pay Back Your Time

Sometimes things get a little out of whack. Say you get to ride all day on your first century (100 miles). Next weekend, make sure more of your time is spent with the people who love and need you. Give your husband a free day from the house to go to a ballgame all day with his buddies.

If you can't balance the time, try a nice night out to dinner, some flowers, or another special way of letting them know how much you appreciate them and the extra effort they give to help you spend time on two wheels. Keep giving as much as you get and your cycling, as well as your life, will be better for it.

CHAPTER 40

Recovery

FOR EVERY WORD EVER WRITTEN ABOUT TRAINING, THERE are half as many about recovery. Rest is as essential to building your strength and endurance as the actual ride. When you exercise, your muscle tissue gets small microtears that when rebuilt make your stronger. The key is, they have to have enough time to rebuild before you beat them up again.

Also factor in what else is happening in your life. Sometimes it's not that you're riding too much, but that you're riding too much for the amount of *other* stress in your life—like starting a new job, moving, having a baby, etc. If you're riding too much, are too stressed out, or are not getting enough sleep, you will not be able to build your fitness. In fact, you could easily end up becoming injured.

This mostly affects those who jump into cycling whole hog, but even casual cyclists can benefit from optimizing their recovery. This means not riding hard every single ride, but sometimes taking the moment to enjoy riding slow. It also means you may not meet your personal plans or goals. Recovery is the spa day, putting your feet up in your man cave, spending time with your family. It's the important work of *not* working so you can do your best and focus when it's time to put out the effort.

Some warning signs that you're burning out are:

> ➤ Fatigue
> ➤ Achy, tired muscles
> ➤ Workouts feeling harder than normal

➤ Crabbiness and irritability

➤ Depression

➤ Low immunity—catching a lot of colds, etc.

➤ Not feeling very hungry

➤ Elevated morning heart rate

Whatever you do, if you're riding so much that you dread even looking at your bike or are feeling stressed instead of psyched about riding, it's time for a break. That might mean shifting your priorities to reduce stress in other parts of your life to help you balance your energy.

Getting Your Z's

For years we've known that we need to get enough sleep. That's why mom sent you to bed early when you were a kid and why lazy mornings feel so great. But the day you decide to sleep in shouldn't be the only day you get a full night's recharge. If you skimp on your hard-earned rest, it's just as bad as not being hydrated or not eating—or, worse, it can affect you exactly the same as a hangover. Basically, how you feel on the bike will not be nearly as good as you could feel.

With our busy schedules, it's easy to shave off a few minutes here or there from our goals to have 7 to 8 hours of sleep a night. Part of the trick is that if you lie down for 7 hours, between

winding down and your natural sleep cycles, you'll get about 6 hours of actual sleep. To get a full night's rest, you need to be in bed trying to sleep for at least 8 to 9 hours. This is way more than most people even attempt to do.

This is important not just to the road cyclist, but to everyone. It's not just the performance on your bike that suffers, but your mental agility and ability to do everyday tasks. Want to perform better at work? Eat better? Be less susceptible to illness and disease? The answer is simple: Hit the hay like your life depends on it.

Here are some simple changes you can make to help you sleep better.

➤ **Don't drink more than one to two drinks per evening.** Although it might make you feel drowsy, it interferes with your sleep cycle and you won't sleep as soundly.

➤ **Avoid caffeine late in the day.** This is a notorious creator of insomnia and fits of restlessness. Stick with your coffee in the morning, then taper by the afternoon.

➤ **Avoid greasy, spicy, or heavy foods close to when you need to rest.** Eating things that are tough to digest can keep you up.

➤ **Get into a bedtime ritual.** This can mean different things for different people. A great way to wind down is with a book, a shower, or listening to soft music. Maybe this is your time to use your foam roller to massage your tired legs. A nightly ritual signals your body to slow your heart rate and relax, easing you into a restful state.

➤ **Remove distracting electronic devices from your bedroom.** This is essential, but much easier said than done. It's too easy to get sucked into Facebook or checking your e-mail on the phone. What's one more episode of your favorite show on Netflix? It's one less half-hour to hour of sleep you'll be getting. Remove computers, phones, and TVs from your bedroom. If you can't, make it a part of your ritual to turn them off at least a half-hour before you try to sleep.

➤ **Make your environment as comfy as possible.** A good mattress and a room that's not too hot, with as little light and noise as possible, will do the trick. Have a partner who's a night owl? Invest in an eye shade and some ear plugs. It's the little things that make all the difference.

CHAPTER 41

Inspiration

RIGHT NOW YOU MAY BE SUPER MOTIVATED TO GET ON A ROAD bike. Or you may just be playing with the idea and need that extra push to jump on the saddle and get rolling. For many riders, after the newness of a shiny toy wears off, they're in need of some motivation to keep them coming back to the bike.

Riding Buddies

One of the easiest ways to find riding encouragement is to find other people to ride with. Having someone you've agreed to meet gives you incentive to hold your word and not play hooky. Not only that, it's the hands-down best way to learn and perfect better riding skills—especially for more advanced riders.

If like many people you're coming to this sport with friends or relatives who cycle (who therefore may be responsible for getting you into this in the first place), see if they'll take you out for a spin. Beware: This can have great or not-so-hot results. We tend to be the hardest on the ones we love, so if you or your riding buddy is frustrated, it can quickly deteriorate into a passionate disagreement. Don't give up on cycling if you aren't enjoying riding with the one who nudged you to get those silly cycling shorts in the first place.

Find local rides in your area—they're a great place to meet fellow riders and discover people who ride at your pace and style. Most bike shops have a daily or weekly ride, or they can connect you with a group who does. Many areas also have local riding clubs and meet-up groups you can easily access online for more information. Group rides are also great sources for finding people you like to ride with outside the group.

Being new to cycling, it can seem a little overwhelming to head out with more experienced cyclists. Don't let riding with faster riders intimidate you or worry about being too slow, feel guilty, or apologize too much for holding the group back. Always remember, everyone started as a newbie, so when they ride with you they'll likely be expecting to keep your pace. If you try to kill yourself to keep up, the other rider will likely think you *want* to go that pace. Falling behind isn't shameful. It's a signal to the other rider(s) to slow down. If they've agreed to a no-drop ride, they'll be waiting for you up the road a bit. Most cyclists are thrilled to have more people out on bikes and want to help you learn lessons that they might have had to find out the hard way, so they're happy to see you in the mix no matter how fast you go.

At one point or another (but especially when learning), every single cyclist has held someone else back on a ride. It's your first rite of passage. The second rite of passage as a cyclist is to ride with people who are slower than you—because you have finally built up your fitness and are no longer the "slow" kid. By riding with faster riders, instead of thinking of how you're holding

them back, remember you're giving them a generous opportunity to be the "fast" ones for a day.

For now, it's easy to get frustrated with the situation because you "know" they can go faster—but what you don't know is if they may really need the break you're giving them. It may be their recovery day, or perhaps they've been sick or have an injury. Assuming that someone dreads riding with you is only going to end with everyone having less fun. You may be helping your fellow riders by reminding them how far they've come, and by providing a great reminder of why it's important to slow down and enjoy the ride. Someday you'll be the faster one, ushering new cyclists into the fold.

Before you show up, ask questions about the ride. How far will you be going? Is there a no-drop policy so you won't get left behind to fend for yourself? What's the expected pace? Will the other riders be willing to really slow down for you? This will ensure you don't end up in a ride that's way over your head.

When you do find people you enjoy riding with and who seem to enjoy a similar pace or riding style, reach out to them. Everyone loves an invite to ride, and the more you ride together, the more you can grow as cyclists together. Road cycling is a great way to meet people who love life, enjoy the outdoors, and enjoy sharing their passion for two wheels. Lifelong friendships have cemented between pushes of the pedals and sharing the adventure of the road.

Dos and Don'ts of Finding Riding Buddies

DO:

➤ **Ask lots of questions.** It's the best (and fastest) way to learn.

➤ **Find a mix of riding buddies**—some who can push you and some who you can grow along with.

➤ **Communicate your intentions for the ride (distance, pace, etc.) before you take off.**

➤ **Come prepared with tubes, tire levers, and an inflation device**—even if you don't know how to change a flat.

➤ **Have enough water and food for however long you planned on riding.**

➤ **Be flexible.** When you're riding with others, sometimes the unexpected takes place.

➤ **Reach out to other riders to see if they're interested in riding again.** It's nice to find a few people to ride with for variety, and they likely will introduce you to more people.

➤ **Thank anyone you ride with.** Anyone can ride alone, but it takes a little effort to synchronize schedules and riding styles.

DON'T:

➤ **Expect other riders to stick by your side.** If you're riding with someone much faster than you, they may ride ahead and then stop and wait for you—especially on climbs. Unless you've discussed that you want to hang out and chat the entire way, this is a fairly normal way to ride.

➤ **Beat yourself up or feel guilty for not being fast enough.** This will not make the ride more fun or help pushing the pedals seem easier. A positive attitude makes for more enjoyable rides.

➤ **Apologize repeatedly.** If you're a little slower, the other rider likely is prepared to slow their pace or wait for you.

➤ **Get frustrated if you're behind.** Remember, you'll be the one who's waiting for others someday.

Strava

Imagine racing your friends without all of you actually having to be on the road at the same time. Strava is an application for your smart phone that offers many features to track your performance on your rides and compare them to other users by collecting data from your ride (it can be used in conjunction by upload-ing the data from cycling computers you're already using) to accumulate all the statistics from your time on the road. You can then use this info to see how you stack up against your earlier performances, or compare yourself to anyone else who's using Strava where you ride or from a select list of people that you tailor for yourself. Essentially, it's a marvelous tool for competing against yourself and others, or for creating camaraderie within the cycling community.

Better yet, it gives you a great opportunity to push yourself to do a little better than your last ride by giving you a way to race yourself. Each route is broken down into segments, and Strava lets you know when you've hit a personal best time and can rank you compared with other cyclists in the area.

Strava can also be a great resource for finding new routes in your area. You can search for the most popular segments to get ideas for where you might want to ride. Since the app comes with map info (including elevation gains and losses), you can decide if it's a route you want to tackle.

Most new riders find it a very helpful (and free!) way to track how they're doing. Here's what one user had to say when he was starting cycling:

I first started riding about 8 months ago . . . so I'm pretty new to just about everything. A buddy of mine clued me in to Strava, and honestly, if not for it . . . I would likely not be riding today. Sure, there were always a bunch of guys out on the local single-track, but I was new . . . and WAY too timid to try and ride with anyone, so I rode all by myself, just me and Strava. Was I racing for a top time? Nope. Am I KOM [King of the Mountain, a racing term for who gets to the top first] of anything? Nope. But was it a valuable "tool" to use to keep me going, YES! Every time I would show up for a ride, I would fire up Strava with the intent to better

my time. It kept me going strong, and more importantly, it kept me interested in biking! Nowadays, I don't use Strava too often since I have gained the confidence and ability to ride with other people, but anytime I'm out for a ride by myself, I just can't help but fire it up, and see just how much improvement I have made . . . over myself!

—Benjamin Rivers (former cycling newbie)

Benjamin used Strava as a stepping-stone to gain confidence and boost his fitness. When used properly, Strava is a great tool for tracking how you're progressing. Keep in mind that although Ben claimed he was scared to ride with others, he got his tip on Strava from a "buddy" who was in the know. This app is not meant to be a replacement for interacting with other cyclists. In fact, it offers a great opportunity to tap into your area's cycling community. If you notice another cyclist who is ranked close to you, send him a message and see if he'd like to ride. If they're on Strava, it's likely they are a little competitive, and you could find someone to push you on actual rides together.

One word of warning: Strava is meant to be used as motivation and friendly competition. Use your head and don't push yourself so hard for new records that you lose sight of the road around you. In their fervor to break records, some cyclists have been injured because the goal became more important than personal safety. Don't let this happen to you!

PART X

TUNING YOUR RIDE

Many of us can be guilty of neglect. You pay a lot for a bike and it's a finely tuned machine, so it should last, right? Much like getting your car's oil changed or fluids flushed, your new bike lasts longer and runs better if you maintain it. This starts with your regular maintenance and includes knowing when to bring it to the experts for repairs.

It's also extremely helpful to know what to do in case of an on-the-road emergency (like a flat tire) and all the little things you should be carrying with you when you head out.

CHAPTER 42

Basic Maintenance 101

MAINTENANCE: SUCH A DREARY WORD. IT MAKES US THINK OF the handyman, the super, the janitor—the guy you call to clean up the mess or fix what's broken. You don't know how to do it so you call someone else. Plus it just seems like it takes way too long. Maybe you don't think of yourself as very mechanically inclined. Besides, if you're already crunched for ride time, how are you supposed to care for your bike, too?

Basic maintenance, in actuality, can be really quick, fun, and easy, as well as help you get to know your bike much better so you have more control over how it rides. By taking care of your bike, it will become less of a mystery machine beneath you and more of a trusty tool you wield to get you where you want to go. Not to mention that maintaining your bike is a huge money saver. By taking care of your ride, you won't need as many expensive parts or repairs in the future.

At the very least, riders need to know how to clean the frame, air up the tires, clean the rims, and clean and oil the chain. These are the very basics of what you should be doing to care for your bike. By mastering them, you'll be empowered to take on any ride, anytime. We'll also give you some big tips on changing flats and how to make the most of your local bike shop so when you do head in for repairs, it's with a smile.

Tire Inflation

Getting your tires aired up properly is the single most important thing you can do to make sure you have a good ride. It's a little like the Goldilocks fable: too much and you'll lose traction; too little can cause flats; somewhere in the middle is always best. To start, you'll need to have a good floor pump with an accurate gauge, which you can buy at your local bike shop, so you know how much air you're putting in.

In the United States, inflation is measured in psi (pounds per square inch) units. The amount your tire needs will usually be printed as a range on the side of the tire—sometimes into the rubber, where it's a little hard to find. It will often read something like 80 psi min.–110 psi max. (5.5 bar–7.6 bar). This tells you the minimum and maximum recommended pressure (the "bar" measurement is a European standard).

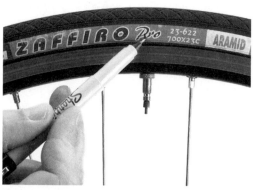

The recommended maximum psi is printed into the side of your tire, as is the tire size.

As a general rule, the max is for a person who weighs 185 pounds or more. If you weigh less, the tire manufacturer will have different recommended inflations on its website. For example, if a rider weighs 140 pounds on one brand of tire, she would inflate her tires to 95 psi in the back and 85 psi in the front. Because more of your weight is on the saddle and centered over the back wheel, you should inflate the front a little less. Since the front wheel controls your steering, using a slightly lower pressure than your rear (by about 10 psi) gives improved traction for better control on turns and descents.

The valve stem is where you put the air into the tube. There are two kinds of stems: One is called Presta, the other Schrader. (See photo in Chapter 4, page 29.)

Most road bikes come with Presta valves, which are skinny and metal with a little nubbin at the top that needs to be unscrewed to let air in or out. Practice depressing this to let air out. You'll sometimes need to do this to prime the valve to let air in, too. Always have the valve stem facing down (between the 10 o'clock and 2 o'clock position) on your wheel to clamp your hose on. Having it there will make it easier to control and give you better positioning for removal of the pump head after inflation. When it's full to the recommended pressure, unclamp the hose and, with both thumbs on the face of the head, push it gently toward the hub at the center of the wheel. You should hear a small gasp of air leave the hose after it's depressurized. If you wiggle the hose or pull it to the side to remove it, you're more than likely to release air from the tube or break the valve stem off.

Because the tube inside the tire is just a big, high-pressure balloon, it usually loses air over a few days to a week. Check your tires every 2 to 3 days, or if you're riding less often, pump them every time you leave for a ride.

Cleaning: Getting Rid of the Grime

The Chain

If you're regularly oiling the chain, you shouldn't have to clean it every time you oil it. Save cleaning for about every 500-plus miles when you can also clean your chainrings (gears in front) and cassette (gears in back). The important thing to remember is that your chain needs lubrication, so overcleaning it can actually wear it out.

Start by flipping your bike upside-down and spraying degreaser (409, a citrus degreaser) or a bike-specific chain cleaner (like the degreaser from WD-40 Bike) on the links and scrubbing with an old toothbrush. After you've lifted most of the dirt, wipe it clean with a rag—unless it's the WD-40 Bike brand degreaser, which you rinse with water. If you've used a spray degreaser directly on the chain, you need to wait 24 hours before applying oil to give time for the degreaser

to evaporate completely from between the links.

There are also gadgets on the market to clean your chain, but the toothbrush-and-degreaser method works just as well. If your chain is only lightly dirty or you want to clean it more regularly, you can spray the degreaser on a rag and wipe the chain clean with it. In either case, there's never a need to remove the chain or the wheel. Both will just make the job harder, and breaking the chain apart will only decrease its life.

Always oil your chain afterward. We'll talk more about this in "Lubrication Equals Love," page 230.

If you want to clean the cassette and chainrings as well, this is a great time. The chainrings you can scrub with a brush and degreaser on the bike. To get to the cassette, take your rear wheel off your bike and lay it

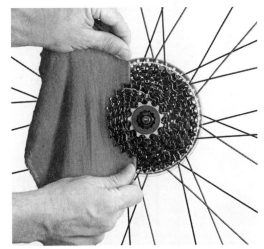

Remove the wheel and lay it with the gears faceup to floss between the gears.

down with the gear side facing up. Spray degreaser on the teeth of the cogs and scrub with a firm brush. Get between the gears with a piece of cardboard or specially made gear-cleaning brush. Floss a rag between each gear and roll it back and forth to clean it free of any debris or black grime.

The Rims

A little science lesson: Most rims are commonly made of aluminum. Like steel oxidizing into rust, aluminum also breaks down when it contacts air, but it breaks down into a strange black dust that is kind of like the graphite from your pencil. Every time it's exposed to air, your rim oxidizes, but that same black oxidization dust protects the aluminum underneath from oxidizing more. Unfortunately, every time you use

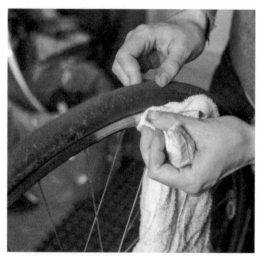

Cleaning your rims is a quick way to extend their life and substantially improve your braking power.

your brakes, you're wiping the old layer off so a new one forms. When it rains, aluminum oxidizes even more and the black grime gets slimy and slippery—which is one of the reasons it's so hard to stop on wet surfaces. If you live anywhere humid or rainy, maintaining your rims is extra important. In the desert or dry areas, it's not as critical, but still nice to maintain.

The easiest way to maintain them regularly is to wipe them down with a dry rag every time you oil the chain (using a different, clean rag, of course), every hundred miles or so. You can also use rubbing alcohol, but avoid using a bottle of spray cleaner or degreaser to get rid of the grunge—it tends to smear around instead of coming off on the rag and leaves a soapy film that can make your brakes squeal. To clean, have your bike upside down and spin the wheel while holding the rag against the braking surface of the rim. It shouldn't take more than 2 minutes to get both sides of the front and rear wheels.

Another option is to clean them while you're cleaning the frame (see the next section). Although a spray cleaner makes a smeary mess, a bucket of soapy dishwater and a firm brush use enough fluid to lift the oxidized dust and let it run off the rim. This method cleans a little deeper than just wiping with a dry rag or rubbing alcohol—just make sure to rinse after soaping up.

The bottom line is, if you don't clean them on a regular basis, the grit will build up—making it much harder to stop, which will make you squeeze the brake harder, which creates even more of the oxidization grit, which will in turn wear the rim out faster. Since the wheels are one of the most expensive parts of your bike, it's a time (not to mention a life) saver that can also help your pocket book.

The Frame

Like with your body, everything feels better and the world is a better place after a nice shower. In the case of your bike, it doesn't have

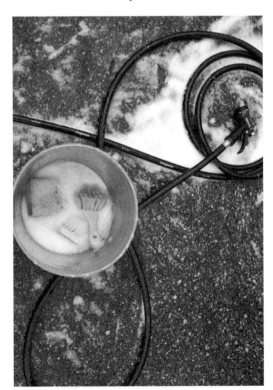

Wash your bike in an upright position and use a gentle stream of water.

to be warm, but a shower is the best because it's the fastest, easiest, and most thorough way to a clean bike. By getting rid of all the road grit, sugary drink drips, and salty sweat, you'll end up with a nicer ride.

You'll need:

➤ A hose (or shower if you don't have an outside hose and can stomach bringing your bike into the bathroom)

➤ A bucket of warm, soapy dishwater

➤ A large, soft sponge like one used for washing a car

➤ A handheld, large-surfaced, medium-bristled car-washing brush and a smaller dishwashing brush

➤ Rubber gloves

Start by rinsing your upright bike gently with the hose or shower to loosen the grime. The keyword is *gentle*. Don't use a strong spray or worse, or you'll risk ruining your bike's bearings by forcing water and dirt where only grease belongs; if you flip your bike over, all the water will run inside the frame. A good rule of thumb for washing your bike is to think of the water pressure as if it's coming out of a watering can.

Use the soapy sponge to clean your frame (the brush might scratch the paint or clear coat). The brush is great for scrubbing off all the black oxidization grime from the rims and getting into harder-to-reach nooks and crannies—like in your brake arms or derailleurs.

Rinse the soap off after cleaning. If you've used the WD-40 Bike brand degreaser mentioned earlier, this is a great time to rinse that off, too. If you didn't, wipe any excess water off the chain so it doesn't rust. When you're finished, pick up your bike a few inches off the ground and drop it a few times to help shake off the water.

You can also use a bottle of spray cleaner or degreaser (409, Simple Green, Citrasolve, or other citrus degreasers work great) and some rags following similar directions, but the shower method works better and cuts your cleaning time by half.

For a nice finishing touch, you can use furniture polish or some specially made bike products that protect the paint on your frame. It not only looks sweet, but it also keeps dirt from accumulating as quickly between cleanings.

Lubrication Equals Love

There are a lot of moving parts on your bike, but nothing gets put through the ringer like your chain. You're entirely dependent on it to make your bike move forward, so it's working constantly with every push of the pedals. If you take a close look at the chain, you'll notice it has plates on the sides, and little rollers in the middle with pins through them holding it all together. When you lubricate your chain,

you're trying to get oil into all the little parts inside of it where metal meets metal to help it move effortlessly.

The most common problems are:

➤ **You don't oil your chain enough (or at all).**
➤ **You put way too much oil on.**

Both of these can cause your chain to wear out before its time—though not oiling your chain is the worst thing you can do. Your chain needs lubrication inside it to flex over all those gears smoothly. If it's dry, it has to work harder to do its job—which creates resistance when you push the pedals. You'll know when this happens, as it will start making a lot of noise that starts to sound like a gentle swishing with each pedal stroke and progresses to a loud, squeaky, creak. One easy trick to getting faster with less effort: Oil your chain every hundred miles—or more often if you get caught (or ride regularly) in the rain.

Too much oil on the chain is like grease on your stove—it collects dirt and makes a mess that's difficult to clean up. Unfortunately, not only will it spatter a black, greasy film all over your frame and wheels (which, as you might guess, doesn't help with stopping), the goopy, greasy dirt will work into those little spaces you're trying to lubricate, wearing down your chain.

Luckily, oiling it is one of the simplest, easiest tasks to do—even for a complete novice. So every hundred miles, here's what to do to keep your chain quiet and give it a nice, long life.

1. Flip your bike over. Your rear wheel will have to be off the ground to run the chain both backward and forward.

2. Where the chain is exposed and not wrapped around any gears, hold the straw or tip of the oil bottle against the chain and turn the pedals five or six times until you've gone around the chain at least twice. Pedal smoothly and at a moderate pace so the oil skims over the top of the chain and spreads out. Don't put a drop of lube on every link—that's a surefire way to over-oil it. Also avoid putting oil on the gears.

3. Wipe the excess lubricant off. While holding a pedal to keep the chain from moving, wrap a rag around an exposed part of your chain and wipe back and forth on the top and bottom until the chain looks clean and free of oil on the outside surface. Work in small sections until you've gone around the chain completely. Don't just run the chain through a rag while pedaling; instead, really scrub the excess oil (and dirt) off the outside of the chain.

4. Work your way around until the entire chain looks clean and there's little to no visible oil or dirt on the outside. This is the most important part of oiling the chain. You need to spend two to three times longer to wipe it down than it took you to put the oil on. This method uses the excess lubricant you've applied to help clean any accumulated dirt or old oil off your chain—like a two-in-one shampoo/conditioner combo!

CHAPTER 43

Tools You Can Use

THERE ARE A LOT OF NIFTY TOOLS OUT THERE TO DO EVERY level of maintenance and repair under the sun. But bike shops have the big tools (and knowledge) so you don't have to. A point in time may come when you want to learn how to do all the work on your own bike, but for now let's stick to the basics. There are tools you'll want to have at home to help with small repairs and routine basic maintenance. On the road you'll want a lighter, more compact version so you don't get stranded on your ride. Even if you don't know how to use them, you never know who might be able to come to your rescue—as long as you have the tools to make the fix.

Home Tools to Keep You Rolling

Truthfully, as you're starting road biking, you don't need much. But what you do need is pretty close to necessity.

> **Floor Pump:** This is a full-size pump that can quickly fill your tires to the proper pressure. Most come with options for both Schrader and Presta valves (see "Tire Inflation," page 226), though the Presta is more commonly

found on most road bikes. Be sure to purchase one with a pressure gauge so you know how much you're filling up the tires and can get a sense of how much they lose between fillings.

› **Tire Levers:** These are your helpers for getting a tire off a rim so you can change a flat. One of the most used tools in a home bike shop.

› **Bottle of Chain Lube:** The only way to keep your chain moving well

› **Degreaser:** For keeping your chain clean and your frame wiped down

› **Rags:** Essential for cleaning chains, rims, and the inevitable spill

› **Screwdrivers:** To add or remove accessories

› **Crescent Wrench:** Not the finest-tuned instrument, but versatile and gets the job done

› **"Y" or Tri 4-5-6mm Hex Tool:** Most of the bolts on your bike are going to be one of these three sizes, as are water bottle cages and other accessories. This inexpensive tool gives you the three most common sizes with the benefit of better leverage than a travel-sized multitool.

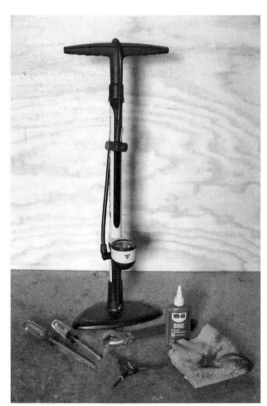

Here's all the tools you need to get started at home: a floor pump, tire levers, chain oil, rags, screwdrivers, a crescent wrench, and a 4-5-6mm "Y" hex tool.

Tools for Your Ride

What you need to carry on the bike is essentially pocket-sized versions of what you have at home. You may not know how to use it all, but it's still important to have it on you. The rider or driver who pulls over to help you on the side of the road can bring the skills—but you'd better back it up with the right tools. These include:

YOUR BASIC ON-THE-ROAD TOOLS

› **Tire Levers**

› **A Patch Kit:** For repairing punctured tubes

› **Multitool:** Includes hex wrenches and screw drivers

› **Inflation Device:** A hand pump or CO_2 inflator

YOUR DELUXE TOURING OR LONG SOLO RIDE TOOLS

➤ **Chain Breaker:** For repairing

➤ **Tire Boot**

➤ **Chain Links or Chain Pins**

➤ **Duct Tape**

➤ **Presta to Shrader Valve Stem Adaptor:** Helps in a pinch if your pump breaks and you need to borrow one that may not have a Presta head on the pump

Note: For a more detailed list of everything else you should carry, see "Bringing Up the Rear" on page 96.

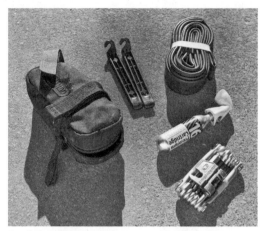

Here's the minimum of what you would carry in your pockets or underseat bag: tire levers, a patch kit, a multi-tool, and an inflation device.

CHAPTER 44

To Serve and Protect: How to Arm Yourself Against Flats

FLAT TIRES ARE HANDS-DOWN THE MOST COMMON BIKE repair, but nobody likes getting a puncture. At best it cuts into your riding time or slows down a group ride; at worst it instills sheer panic in riders who don't feel confident in their ability to get back on the road. The good news is that there are quite a few things you can do to protect against flats so that you're a lot less likely to get them in the first place.

Protect

Buying puncture-resistant tires is your best line of defense, period. Many of today's tires come with a Kevlar liner that makes it harder for little objects to sneak through

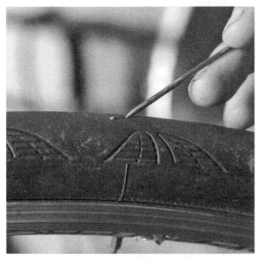

Kevlar built into the tire keeps debris from getting through—even a piece of glass or metal that's still stuck in the tread.

your tread and ruin your ride. The thicker the puncture resistance, the heavier the tire, so you'll have to decide how much protection you want versus how much extra weight you want to carry. If you're a racer who wants a lighter-weight training tire, you might go with a little less protection. On a bike tour where you'll be hauling extra weight anyway, fewer flats and heavier tires might be the better choice. Luckily, there are a lot of middle-ground options so you can get a good barrier from the road without bogging down your ride too much.

Most people should avoid self-sealing, slime-filled tubes and tire liners. Both are heavier and more trouble than they are worth, *unless* you live where cacti and desert thorns are an issue, and then they can become absolute life-savers. In those situations, it can mean the dif-ference between being stranded after your fourth flat in the hot sun or having a ride free of any mishaps.

It's also good to make sure your tires are properly inflated before your ride. A tire that's too low can cause something called a "pinch" flat where your tube gets caught between your rim and tire when you hit a pothole or rock. The more you weigh, the bigger this problem will be—so a 110-pound woman is not nearly as likely to experience pinch flats as a 225-pound man. This is easily avoided with a quick pressure check before you head out the door.

Replace your tires when the tread is flat, has a lot of cuts in it, or if the sidewall is showing wear. Your rear tire is going to wear out first because your weight is over it. Don't think you can just swap front and rear, though. If your rear tire tread has flattened out from wear and you put it on the front, you're going to be up on a corner when you lean into a turn—which is bad news for stability. If you put the less-worn front on the rear, you're going to need a new tire sooner than later anyway. It's easiest (and a nicer ride) to replace both when the rear is worn.

Plan Wisely

Always have at least one spare tube, a patch kit, and an inflation device (pump or CO_2) with you. Not having to patch the tube on the side of the road will make things faster. The side of your tire will tell you what size tube you need. The patch kit is still an excellent backup in case of multiple flats. Also, carry tire levers and some kind of boot in case the hole in your tire is so big it needs to be repaired as well. A foot length of duct tape in your seat pack is always handy, but a dollar bill or a thick energy-bar wrapper can both work in a pinch.

Tube Talk: How to Choose the Right Size

Tubes come in many different sizes and valve stem lengths, and you'll need to have the right one on hand when the time comes to fix your flat.

Tube Size

First, look at the side of your tire for a series of numbers that start with 700c (or less commonly, and usually found on small bikes, 650b).

It will be followed by an "x" and a second number. The first number is how big your wheel is around, and the second number is how wide that particular tire is. Most road bikes will be somewhere between 23c and 28c, except for touring bikes, which are sometimes wider.

So your tire will usually read something like this:

700 x 23c

700 x 25c

700 x 28c

Pump, Pump It Up

CHOOSE YOUR INFLATION DEVICE WISELY, AND PRACTICE using it once before you hit the road.

CO_2

Pro: Super quick if speed is your priority.

Con: You're limited to the number of cartridges you can carry. After that it's cell phone city. Also, it can be as heavy or heavier than a lightweight pump.

LIGHTWEIGHT HAND PUMP

Pro: Lighter than any other option and small enough not to add grams to your ride if you're counting. Some come with a hose for easy use.

Con: Depending on design, your arms may tire before you hit the inflation you want. No bells or whistles here.

TOURING HAND PUMP

Pro: Can come with a gauge, foot stops, and lots of bells and whistles. Easily attaches to your bike either on a frame mount or under a water bottle cage. Designed to be easy.

Con: These are the heaviest and bulkiest of inflation devices by far, often taking up valuable space and not easily packed down.

The tube will follow the same number series, except that because tubes are basically fancy balloons, the box will read a range like this:

700 x 20–28c

700 x 28–34c

If your tire falls anywhere inside the given range, the tube will fit. In a pinch, you can always use a narrower tube in a wider tire (for example, a 28c at the top range will fit into a 34c tire). However, you can't stuff a bigger tube into a smaller tire (a 34c tube will not work in a 25c tire).

Valve Length

Valves come in three main lengths depending on how deep your rim is. Your wheel's rim used to be kind of square, but for aerodynamic purposes has become a little more triangular (called a "v" rim). This means that your tube needs a valve stem that's a little longer to be able to have enough of it sticking out to get the pump head securely on when you inflate it. You can always use a stem that's too long, but if it's too short, you're out of luck.

The most common length needed for road bikes is now 48mm. It's the middle length and will fit most "v" rims.

The old standard is 32mm. It's usually too short to work on modern rims, but is sometimes okay for touring rims (which tend to be beefier and less concerned with aerodynamics) or older rims.

There's also 64mm, an extra-long valve for very deep "v" rims, usually found on time-trial bikes.

If you're not sure which one you need, bring your bike or wheel into the bike shop with you.

CHAPTER 45

Becoming a Flat-Repair Pro

IT'S A BEAUTIFUL DAY, YOU'RE TIRED FROM RIDING—OR JUST heading out, or trying to sneak in a quick spin before the sun goes down—and *BAM*. *Psssss*. Flat city.

No one has any love for the annoyance, the waste of precious ride time, or, in some cases, the end to your ride. For the average rider, it's a 10- to 15-minute detour that ceases your ride momentum. If you don't know how to change a flat, it's a complete game changer, leaving you subject to the fates of riders or drivers around you—or a desperate cell phone call.

No matter who you are, flats are one of the more involved repairs on a bike. Most riders (and mechanics) think flats are an easy fix and that if you don't know how to do it, you're somehow lacking in character, or not a "real" cyclist. Wrong. Sure, they're easy—after you've had hundreds of them or if you're a mechanic who changes them 10 times a day.

Don't let this stop you from learning how. You can become a skilled flat-repair expert—even if you barely know how to use a screwdriver and call your brother for any home emergency. We're going to talk you through it and key you in to all the little tips and tricks that most mechanics and lifetime cyclists know—yet usually forget to mention when they try to show you how in a 5-minute quick demo. These are the nitty-gritty details that can cut minutes off your repair time and give you the confidence you need to journey out as far and wide as you can dream.

So when a flat tire does happen, you'll be eager for the chance to try out your new repair skills. Practice, practice, practice (at least three times in a row your first time) and it will be a breeze. Onward: boldly, bravely, and confidently.

YOU'LL NEED:

➤ A new tube

➤ 2 tire levers

➤ A floor pump, hand pump, or CO_2 cartridge and inflator

Removing the Wheel

The rear wheel is the most difficult to get off—but also the most likely place for a flat since most of your weight is centered over it.

1. Remove any accessories from your handlebars (such as your computer).

2. Shift into the smallest gear in the rear cluster (closest to the outside of the bike).

3. Release the quick release on your brakes.

4. Flip your bike over.

5. Open the quick release lever (C-shaped lever near the center of the wheel) by flipping the handle open and loosen the nut one turn. Don't take it all the way off, otherwise it's no longer a "quick" release.

6. Take note that the chain is a loop and the rear gear cluster rests inside the loop. You've got to get it out of there. Standing behind the bike, roll the cleanest part of the rear derailleur (the part that the chain goes through near your rear wheel) back by pulling hard on it to make a clear path for the gears to pull away from the chain.

7. Pull the wheel up and out of the bike frame, and lift the chain off the gears.

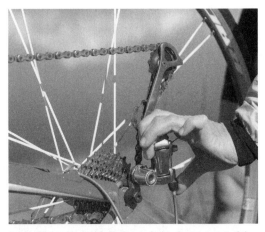

As the bike rests upside down, grab the cleanest part of the rear derailleur from behind the bike and pull it back toward you to make room for the cassette to clear the chain.

TOP TIPS:

➤ Don't be afraid to manhandle your bike to get the wheel off. On some bikes, it will need some less-than-gentle persuasion to pull it from the frame. You won't hurt the bike.

➤ Practice taking the wheel off and putting it back on at least two or three times to get the hang of it. Getting the hang of this alone will take 5 to 10 minutes off your total time.

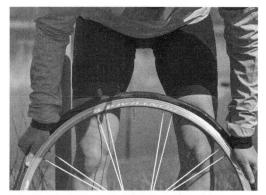

Grab the tread of the tire (but not the rim) with both hands and push any slack to the side that's opposite the valve stem.

Removing the Tire

1. Remove as much air as possible from the tire by compressing the valve stem. Really push every last bit out. Even a tiny amount in the tube will make it much harder to remove the tire.

2. With the wheel resting on the floor and the valve stem near you and facing downward, place your hands on the tread facing out (palms down, fingers facing away from you), grab the sidewalls of the tire between your fingers and thumb, and drag the tire around toward the side of the wheel opposite the valve stem. This will bring any slack from the tire to one area, making it much easier to remove. If you're lucky, you might be able to lift both beads (the edges of the tire that hook into the rim) of the tire up and over the edge of the rim—avoiding the use of tire levers and skipping to step 6.

3. Working at the area opposite the valve stem (where you've conveniently pushed the slack), use a tire lever to scoop one bead over the rim edge and hook the other end of the lever on the spoke below it to hold the lever in place. With the second lever, repeat scooping the bead over the rim, but this time pull the second lever out with each scoop until enough slack is created to make the tire loose enough to easily fit the tire lever under the exposed section of bead.

4. Run the lever around the rim so one bead is entirely off.

5. Remove the tube up to the valve stem.

6. Lift an inch of the second bead (or beads) up and over the edge of the rim, hold the wheel on the ground vertically, then push straight down firmly with your palm toward the ground to remove the tire.

TOP TIPS:

> If you're in a race or a group ride situation, it may be quicker to remove only one bead. Be aware this makes it much tougher to find what caused the puncture.

Finding the Puncture

1. If you're using a pump, overinflate the tube to find where your puncture is. This will help determine what caused your flat.

2. Squeeze the tread of your tire the entire way around to look for debris that may have caused this flat—or some that hasn't worked through the tread yet and may cause a flat later. Remove all debris.

3. Check your rim strip (the piece of cloth or plastic lining on the inside of your rim) to make sure it's firmly in place and no spoke holes are exposed (which can cause flats).

Replacing the Tube and Tire

1. Inflate your new tube very slightly with your hand pump or by mouth if you're using CO_2. You need only a very small amount of air so the sides of the tube are no longer sticking together. Too much air will make getting the tire back on difficult.

2. Put the tube into the tire with the valve stem at the tire label. Bike shops usually do this to help give you a point of reference the next time you have a flat—so when you inflate the tube and find your hole, you'll know exactly where to find the culprit in the tire.

3. With the rim resting on your feet, make sure the whole tire is on one side of the wheel.

4. You'll be putting one side of the tire on at a time. Push the valve stem of the tube through the hole in the rim, making sure the bead closest to your body is sitting inside the rim. The other side of the tire will be hanging off the rim.

5. Starting at the valve stem and working both hands around in a rainbow till they meet on the opposite side, push the entire bead you've started back on the rim. Be sure to check by looking on both sides of the wheel that the first bead is entirely on.

6. Start back to the valve stem to get the second side of the tire on. With your left hand about an inch over from the valve stem, pinch and hold the remaining bead toward the middle of the rim but *do not* tuck it entirely into the rim. At the same time, with your right hand start a few inches over to the right of the valve stem and work the same bead into the rim until it begins to settle in.

7. After the bead starts to tuck into the rim, work both hands around the rim in opposite directions (like a rainbow on

each side), pressing on the sidewall to tuck as much of the bead as you can until you are opposite the valve stem. Important: Make sure the tube is tucked into the rim well and not pinching between the bead and rim edge as you tuck the tire in. Usually by the time you reach opposite the valve stem, there will be one part of the tire left that's not easy to get over the edge of the rim.

➤ Tip: Push on the side of the tire instead of the bead to push it on to the rim. This provides better leverage.

8. To get the final bit of tire over, start with both hands very close to each other and wrap them around one of the edges that won't easily go over. With your thumb under the rim and your hand wrapped around the tire, twist the tread of the tire over the edge of the rim away from you, pulling the remaining bead over the edge. This is called the "gorilla grip" because you're focused on using the palm of your hand as opposed to pushing on the bead with your thumb.

➤ Tip: The gorilla grip is very similar to what you might have done as a kid to torture your brother, sister, or cousin by wrapping both hands around their forearm right up next to each other and then twisting their skin back and forth. Use the same grip around the rim as you would on their arm (thumbs wrapped

underneath). Then, instead of moving your hands in opposite directions, roll them both toward the side you want the tire to go onto.

9. If the gorilla grip doesn't work, use the tire lever to get the remainder of the tire on the rim. Warning: Using tire levers to get the bead onto the rim is a common cause of pinch flats. You can cause a flat by using tire levers to put the bead on, so be careful.

10. When you're down to 4 inches or less of bead left to put on the rim, try the gorilla grip again.

11. Push the valve stem into the tire to make sure it's moving freely. If not, you may have gotten the tube caught under the bead near the valve stem. Double-check before proceeding. If it's caught, remove one side of the tire, go back to step 5, and try again.

Inflating the Tire

1. On the tire above the valve stem, pinch the sidewalls together to force the stem firmly out and make it easier to put the pump head or CO_2 inflator on.

2. Inflate to around 20 psi. Check that the edge of the tire is seated into the rim properly. If it's bulging or you can see the bead, deflate, check to make sure the tube isn't caught under the edge of the tire, press the bead into the rim, and inflate again to check for bulging.

3. Inflate to your recommended psi. Remember the max psi (printed on the side of your tire) is for a person who weighs over 185 pounds (84 kg). If you weigh less, the tire manufacturer will have different recommended inflations on its website. For example, for someone who weighs 140 pounds (63.5 kg) should inflate his or her tires to 95 psi (6.5 bars) in the back and 85 psi (5.9 bars) in the front. (It's typical to use less in the front because less of one's weight is over it, offering improved traction on turns and descents).

Reinstalling the Wheel

1. Standing behind the bike, find your loop and chain and place the gears inside the loop, resting the smallest, most outside gear of the wheel on the piece of chain closest to the derailleur.

2. As you did during removal, stand at the back of your overturned bike and pull the clean part of the derailleur back to make a clear path for the gears to get past it and into the frame. (See photo on page 240.)

3. Push the wheel down toward the seat of the bike to get it down past the derailleur.

4. Push the wheel back and down toward your feet until it sits on the frame.

5. Make sure the wheel looks straight in the frame.

6. Close your quick release on your wheel.

➤ Tip: Overtightening the quick release can damage your wheel and make it harder for your bike to move forward. Tighten firmly, but not so hard you'd need two hands to open it later. It has been designed not to be overtightened. Also, don't close the lever against the frame, but rather next to it—against and it not only may not be closed all the way, but also will be hard to get your fingers behind to open it next time.

7. Flip the bike back over and close the quick release on your brakes.

8. Remember to take your old tube with you, and don't leave any trash or tools behind. Always carry a patch kit in case you have more than one flat in one ride.

CHAPTER 46

Service Guide: When to Head to the Shop (and Why)

Annual Maintenance

It's important to keep to a regular maintenance schedule, mainly because if you don't take care of your bike, it's going to fall to pieces. How can this machine worth thousands of dollars break down? It can happen the same way your kitchen knife gets dull. You use it a lot . . . and then it gets dangerous and potentially more expensive to fix. As many cyclists can tell you, letting things go too long can cause greater damage to both you and your bicycle in the long run, from unexpected failure of parts to worn-out bits creating worse problems and costing more. It's just like changing the oil in a car so you won't have to replace the engine. Ultimately, this will help save you some heartache and money.

Winter is a great time to go in for service because most shops run discounts and you'll have your bike back in no time due to their lighter workload. Often in the spring and summer, mechanics are juggling helping customers at the counter, answering the phone, and working on a repair. This makes the off-season the best time if you want the best-quality work possible—but really, any time of year you give your bike a little love is a good time!

Here's a list of common services and parts and when you might need them. You can always get service done "à la carte" (or bit by bit as needed), but it's usually more expensive than getting it all done during a tune-up or overhaul.

Tune-Up

Should happen once every year (about every 1,000 to 2,000 miles). Includes a light cleaning, cable adjustments, brake pad replacement, light lubrication, wheel truing, and bearing adjustments. Parts are extra, and most often installation for parts is extra, too. Runs about $80 in labor.

Overhaul

Should happen once ever year (about 2,000-plus miles; every other year if you're riding lightly or using more than one bike). Includes disassem-bling the bike for a deep cleaning; replacing/re-greasing hubs, headsets, and bottom brackets; cleaning your cranks, cassette, chain, and derailleurs; changing cables or other parts if needed; bar tape replacement; and a complete tune-up. Parts are always extra, but most installation is included. Runs about $250 in labor but is often closer to $125 in the winter.

Tires

Usually will need to be replaced every 1,000 to 2,000 miles, depending on type and riding conditions. Common signs of tires in need of replacement are cuts or slits, getting two to three flats in less than a month, and the tread of the tire getting worn down from round to flat (usually more evident in the rear). Do not be tempted to just swap the front and rear tires!

Brake Pads

These may need to be changed more than once a season. Look for the wear indicator lines and feel for the brake lever reaching close to the handlebar as signs that they may need to be replaced.

Cables

If they have more than 3,000 miles or are feel-ing gummy or tight, or the brake or shifter lever isn't returning correctly, it may be time for new cables. Always replace housing with cables.

Chain

Every 1,500 to 2,000 miles, depending on rider weight, strength, and riding style. The chain wears with the cassette, so changing (and lubing) your chain often is the best way to get the most out of the rest of your drivetrain. Measure with a ruler from pin to pin. If at 1 foot there is more than $\frac{1}{16}$-inch stretch, you need a new chain.

Cassette

If the chain has worn too much, or you have been through multiple chains on one cassette (usually two to three), it's time to replace the cassette. Try running your fingernail along the back edge of the teeth to check for wear. If it catches, you may need a new cassette.

Bearing Adjustments

If something on your bike feels "jangly," "loose," or "wiggly," it may be a bearing that needs to be adjusted. For wheels, grab the rim at the top and wiggle left and right; for bottom brackets, grab each crank and wiggle toward the frame (don't grab the pedals!); for headsets, grab the front brake lever and rock the bike front to back a few times. If you feel ticking when you do any of these, the bearing may need adjustment. Riding a bearing out of adjustment may cost more to fix the longer it goes unadjusted. This usually is checked in a tune-up and completely re-lubricated in an overhaul.

CHAPTER 47

Getting the Most from Your Local Bike Shop

Q *Which is the best bike shop in town?*

A **The one that treats you like they want your business and are as passionate about your ride experience as they are about theirs.**

Whether you are buying a bike, bringing it in for a tune-up, or just dropping in for a new tube, your shop should be happy to see you. Most local bike shops are fine establishments working hard to bring you the best service possible to keep you on your bike. Like any relationship, it's a give-and-take situation. If you invest in their knowledge, know-how, and expertise by spending your money there, you should get great customer service in return.

First and foremost, expect to be treated with respect. You shouldn't have to be a lifetime friend of the shop owner or on their racing team to get quality service. You should feel free to ask questions. It's their job to be the experts, so don't be afraid to ask anything, even what you might consider a "stupid question." The more you understand your bike, the better your experience will be. The number one goal of a quality shop is for you to have a good time while you're on your bike—whether that's commuting, touring, or racing.

If you feel that the mechanic or salesperson is being condescending or unhelpful, don't just walk out. Try talking with management first. Most shops (at least the good ones) really want and need feedback to make everyone's experience better. If that doesn't get results, choose another shop.

That being said, also be sure to tell management or owners when you have an excellent experience. Bike shop employees are not in it for the money but are more likely motivated by their love of bikes. A few kudos go a long way on a busy summer day. On that note, it's also a welcome idea to tip your mechanics. They often go above and beyond to get you back on the road and usually get paid less than your average restaurant worker or barista. If you'd tip someone in the service industry for making coffee or pouring a drink, why not extend the same thanks to your mechanic whose hard work can—no exaggeration—save your life?

In the summertime, shops are slammed with business. If you know your bike needs work or an annual tune-up, be prepared—they may be 2 weeks or more out on major repairs. You may also have to wait a bit longer for help from a salesperson or to get rung up at the counter. Have a little extra patience.

If you can, plan ahead a bit for your annual service. Many bicycle shops run service specials in the winter—no wait and a major discount. It also pays off to register for their e-newsletters or e-mail updates. Some shops will even have sales, rides, classes, and special events that you'll be privy to.

As for the classes, if you're intimidated for your first flat change or want to learn more about what products your local shop recommends, classes are great opportunities to ask lots of questions in a more interactive setting. This is another avenue the shop gives you to make connections and take better care of your bike—often for free—so take advantage of it.

Finally, don't expect to borrow your shop's tools. Some shops will have a loaner set, so it is worth (politely) asking. Don't get offended if they don't lend their personal or shop tools out. They need them to do their jobs, and loaner tools often unintentionally end up walking out of the shop in someone's pocket. If you want to work on projects (like changing brake pads or installing fenders), either do them at home or hire the shop to do it for you. You wouldn't come to a restaurant and ask to use the stove, so have the same respect.

Most bike shops make as little as a 1 percent profit margin. Keep this in mind when you're debating whether to get that awesome online deal or go to your local bike shop. Help them out by being a good patron, and they'll be around for the long haul when you have that emergency fix the day before your big ride. You can't say that about an online retailer.

Acknowledgments

I COULD NOT HAVE WRITTEN THIS WITHOUT DANIEL. YOU NOT only filled the book out with your beautiful photography, but held me up with your unending patience and kept me sustained, grounded, well-fed, and exercised as I lost myself in the laptop.

Without my official editors Mark Weinstein, Stephanie Sun, and David Howard, as well as the beautiful and scientifically accurate illustrations from Adam Wallenta, this book would not be nearly as interesting or well worded. The entire nutrition chapter would be a mere wisp without the help of Dr. Stacy Simms, who is single-handedly changing the world of sports nutrition—especially for women.

Many thanks to my unofficial editors and mentors, Desiree and Anne, as well as the guidance and publishing expertise of April Streeter. CD, you know your mojo and your library were essential.

Thanks especially and always to my mom and dad. They made sure I learned the importance and magic of reading and writing—especially my mom, who volunteered to read books in my school and at the public library when I was a kid. You started me on a lifelong love affair with words, learning, and imagination.

There is a very special place in my heart for my cycling and wrenching students who are always teaching and inspiring me to push my boundaries and remember how exciting and fulfilling the first time can be. Allowing me to help you ride confidently on two wheels—sometimes for the very first time—is a great gift and makes me proud beyond imagination.

About the Author

TEACHING, BICYCLES, AND WRITING ARE TORI BORTMAN'S passions, so it was inevitable she would combine them into one career. While learning mechanics and riding skills from the ground up as an adult, she became frustrated trying to find good teachers who understood that bike skills—whether riding, wrenching, commuting, or racing—can be daunting. Dissatisfied, she vowed that it would be her job to make repairing and riding bicycles accessible to anyone, no matter how "mechanically inclined" or "graceful" they claimed not to be. After becoming a professional mechanic, this inspiration led her to start her own bicycle maintenance, skills programs, and corporate consulting business, Gracie's Wrench. Through Gracie's Wrench, she now offers regular courses and workshops covering everything from flat repair to tune-ups to wheel building, plus consulting services for businesses that are ready to make their environment more bike friendly. Her international freelance writing career includes regular contributions to *Bicycle* magazine, *Privateer* magazine, and cycling-focused websites. She resides in Portland, Oregon, with her better half, Daniel, and their adorable and snuggly adopted pit-bull mutt, Memphis (who loves bikes as much as they do).

Index

Boldface page references indicate illustrations or photographs. <u>Underscored</u> references indicate boxed text.

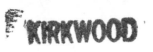